T0335971

New Directions in Geriatric Medicine

Lee Ann Lindquist

Editor

New Directions
in Geriatric Medicine

Concepts, Trends,
and Evidence-Based Practice

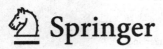
Springer

Editor
Lee Ann Lindquist
Division of General Internal Medicine
  and Geriatrics
Northwestern University Feinberg School
  of Medicine
Chicago, IL, USA

ISBN 978-3-319-28135-3   ISBN 978-3-319-28137-7   (eBook)
DOI 10.1007/978-3-319-28137-7

Library of Congress Control Number: 2016934408

© Springer International Publishing Switzerland 2016
This work is subject to copyright. All rights are reserved by the Publisher, whether the whole or part of the material is concerned, specifically the rights of translation, reprinting, reuse of illustrations, recitation, broadcasting, reproduction on microfilms or in any other physical way, and transmission or information storage and retrieval, electronic adaptation, computer software, or by similar or dissimilar methodology now known or hereafter developed.
The use of general descriptive names, registered names, trademarks, service marks, etc. in this publication does not imply, even in the absence of a specific statement, that such names are exempt from the relevant protective laws and regulations and therefore free for general use.
The publisher, the authors and the editors are safe to assume that the advice and information in this book are believed to be true and accurate at the date of publication. Neither the publisher nor the authors or the editors give a warranty, express or implied, with respect to the material contained herein or for any errors or omissions that may have been made.

Printed on acid-free paper

This Springer imprint is published by Springer Nature
The registered company is Springer International Publishing AG Switzerland

Contents

Contributors

Elizabeth N. Chapman Geriatric Research Education and Clinical Center (GRECC), University of Wisconsin-Madison School of Medicine and Public Health, Madison, WI, USA

Melissa Dattalo Geriatric Research Education and Clinical Center (GRECC), William S. Middleton Memorial VA Hospital, University of Wisconsin-Madison School of Medicine and Public Health, Madison, WI, USA

Linda V. DeCherrie Department of Geriatrics and Palliative Medicine, Mount Sinai Medical Center, New York, NY, USA

Elizabeth Eckstrom Division of General Internal Medicine and Geriatrics, Oregon Health and Science University, Portland, OR, USA

Jennifer Fernandez Division of General Internal Medicine and Geriatrics, Northwestern University Feinberg School of Medicine, Chicago, IL, USA

Maristela Baruiz Garcia Division of Geriatrics, Department of Medicine, David Geffen School of Medicine at UCLA, Los Angeles, CA, USA

Patricia Harris Division of Geriatrics, Department of Medicine, David Geffen School of Medicine at UCLA, Los Angeles, CA, USA

Bobby Heagerty OHSU Brain Institute, Oregon Health and Science University, Portland, OR, USA

Fernanda Heitor Division of General Internal Medicine and Geriatrics, Northwestern University Feinberg School of Medicine, Chicago, IL, USA

Ned Wilson Holland Jr. Division of General Medicine and Geriatrics, Department of Medicine, Emory University School of Medicine, Atlanta Veterans Affairs Medical Center, Decatur, GA, USA

Amy Hsu Division of Geriatrics, Department of Medicine, San Francisco Veterans Affairs Medical Center; University of California, San Francisco, San Francisco, CA, USA

Alison J. Huang Department of Medicine, University of California, San Francisco, San Francisco, CA, USA

Jill Huded Department of Medicine, Louis Stokes Cleveland Veterans Affairs Medical Center, Case Western Reserve University School of Medicine, Cleveland, OH, USA

Geetha Iyer Department of Epidemiology, Johns Hopkins Bloomberg School of Public Health, Baltimore, MD, USA

Ming Jang Division of Geriatrics, Perelman School of Medicine, Hospital of the University of Pennsylvania, Philadelphia, PA, USA

Lee Ann Lindquist Division of General Internal Medicine and Geriatrics, Northwestern University Feinberg School of Medicine, Chicago, IL, USA

Rachel K. Miller Division of Geriatrics, Perelman School of Medicine, Hospital of the University of Pennsylvania, Philadelphia, PA, USA

Emily Morgan Division of General Internal Medicine and Geriatrics, Oregon Health and Science University, Portland, OR, USA

Stephanie Nothelle Department of Medicine, Johns Hopkins Bayview Medical Center, Baltimore, MD, USA

Jennifer Reckrey Departments of Medicine and Geriatrics and Palliative Medicine, Icahn School of Medicine at Mount Sinai, New York, NY, USA

Theresa Rowe Division of General Internal Medicine and Geriatrics, Northwestern University Feinberg School of Medicine, Chicago, IL, USA

Anne M. Suskind Department of Urology, University of California, San Francisco, San Francisco, CA, USA

Quratulain Syed Division of General Medicine and Geriatrics, Department of Medicine, Grady Memorial Hospital, Emory University School of Medicine, Atlanta, GA, USA

Can Dementia Be Delayed? What You Need to Know to Counsel Your Older Patients

Emily Morgan, Bobby Heagerty, and Elizabeth Eckstrom

Patient Scenario

Dr. H is a retired chemist who moved with his wife to the west coast to be closer to his family. When I met him several years ago at age 83, he was vibrant, witty, and a loving husband, father, and grandfather. He and his wife quickly learned to find their way around their new community and settled comfortably into a new life of spending time with family. However, it wasn't long before subtle changes started to occur. Mrs. H noticed that Dr. H was choosing not to go on walks with her. She was interested in getting to know neighbors and attend cultural events in their community, but he preferred to stay home. Within a year or two of meeting Dr. H, it was clear that he had mild cognitive impairment, and now at 88, he is in the early stages of Alzheimer's disease.

Any primary care physician who cares for older adults will recognize this as an all-too-common scenario and has probably agonized over her seeming inability to do anything to prevent it. Nonsteroidal anti-inflammatory drugs, aspirin, estrogen, gingko, and many other drugs have been studied and found to have no impact on cognitive health. We know that medical conditions such as diabetes and stroke predispose to the development of cognitive decline [1] and that cognitive decline comes in all shapes and sizes—from gradually progressive Alzheimer's disease

E. Morgan • E. Eckstrom (✉)
Division of General Internal Medicine and Geriatrics, Oregon Health and Science University,
3181 SW Sam Jackson Park Rd L475, Portland, OR 97239, USA
e-mail: Eckstrom@ohsu.edu

B. Heagerty
OHSU Brain Institute, Oregon Health and Science University,
3181 SW Sam Jackson Park Rd, Portland, OR 97239, USA

© Springer International Publishing Switzerland 2016
L.A. Lindquist (ed.), *New Directions in Geriatric Medicine*,
DOI 10.1007/978-3-319-28137-7_1

(AD) to devastating frontotemporal dementia that may occur at a very young age. But until recently, we had little evidence that anything is effective for delaying or preventing cognitive decline. Fortunately, that is changing. This chapter briefly describes the scope of the problem of cognitive decline, provides some important details about normal brain aging (critical to counseling patients), and then delves into the evidence for diet, exercise, cognitive stimulation, and creative endeavors in reducing risk of cognitive decline. It concludes by offering suggestions for communicating with patients and families about cognitive decline. It is not a comprehensive review but a practical guide that primary care physicians can share with persons of all ages to promote brain health. It does not attempt to synthesize the varied evidence for or against nutritional supplements in healthy brain aging, but will focus on common lifestyle factors that everyone could employ—yet few of us do.

The Scope of the Problem of Cognitive Decline

Alzheimer's disease and related dementias are chronic, debilitating, and fatal diseases that primarily affect individuals 65 and older but surface decades earlier in some patients. Alzheimer's disease is currently the most feared disease of Americans. As baby boomers age, there will be an exponential growth of those with dementia, putting an enormous strain on families, our healthcare system, and the US economy. Dementia is not just a burden for patients and their families but for all of society as bankers, lawyers, drivers, and many others could be cognitively impaired and jeopardize the safety and security of all. It has been called the "defining disease of the boomer generation" and is a public health crisis.

1. Today, over five million Americans are living with Alzheimer's disease and related dementias; by 2050, up to 16 million will have dementia. Dementia is the sixth leading cause of death in the United States. In 2014, the direct costs of caring for those with dementia totaled an estimated $214 billion, including $150 billion in costs to Medicare and Medicaid. By 2050, these costs could rise as high as $12 trillion. Nearly one in every five dollars of Medicare spending is spent on people with Alzheimer's and related dementias. Two-thirds of the five million seniors with Alzheimer's disease are women; women in their 60s are twice as likely to develop Alzheimer's disease over the rest of their lives as they are to develop breast cancer [2].

   More than 15 million Americans provided 17.7 million hours of unpaid care to family members or friends with dementia in 2014 at an estimated cost of $220 billion. Nearly 60 % of dementia caregivers rate the emotional stress of caregiving as high or very high; more than one-third report symptoms of depression. Due to the physical and emotional toll of caregiving, dementia caregivers had $9.3 billion in additional health care costs of their own in 2013 [2].

What Is Normal Cognitive Aging?

Cognition changes throughout the life cycle, and cognitive aging has been defined by a 2015 Institute of Medicine report as "a process of gradual, ongoing, yet highly variable changes in cognitive functions that occur as people get older" [3]. Research on normal physiologic aging of the brain is difficult to accomplish for many reasons. Most studies do not have the length of follow-up needed to discern whether subjects with apparently normal cognitive function at study enrollment will eventually go on to develop mild cognitive impairment or a major neurocognitive disorder. In those that are true longitudinal studies, drop outs tend to be the least healthy "normal" adults, which can lead to confounding. Enrollment bias may also be an issue, as studies on aging may draw healthier, more robust older adults to volunteer. Despite these limitations, researchers are attempting to understand what differentiates inevitable neurocognitive changes that are a result of the aging process from neurocognitive diseases that can be prevented or treated.

At the cellular level, white matter volume begins to decrease at age 40. The largest volume changes are seen in the corpus callosum, which affects the ability of brain's hemispheres to communicate [4]. In comparison, there is minimal change in gray matter volume with aging, though a few specific areas such as the cerebellum do show localized volume loss. The white matter loss is due to changes in neuronal structures which cause an overall decreased ability to complete nerve signal propagation, resulting in slowed retrieval and response times in various areas of the brain. In fact, signal transmission in the central nervous system is seen to decrease a few milliseconds per year starting as young as age 20 [5–7]. While a specific pattern of volume loss is seen in normal aging, atrophy in Alzheimer's disease is also not random. Atrophy in AD usually evolves slowly, following a pathway that first involves the entorhinal cortex and the hippocampus, and then spreads out to associated areas in the medial parietal, lateral temporal, and frontal regions, eventually affecting all regions of the cortex. This organized pattern of atrophy in early AD can be used to differentiate between low and high risk of progression to AD in non-demented or elderly individuals [8].

Study of axonal and synaptic changes with aging has led to the "last in, first out" hypothesis, which postulates that areas of the brain which are last to differentiate in neurodevelopment produce thinner myelin, leaving them more susceptible to deterioration with aging [7]. Primary motor and visual areas are the first to fully myelinate in neurodevelopment, and these processes are preserved in healthy aging. Frontal and temporal association areas are the last to myelinate in the developing brain. It is these more complex neural networks that underlie higher cognitive functions such as memory, executive functions, and language which start to deteriorate with normal aging. Along with structural changes, we also see age-related changes in neurotransmitters such a dopamine. Reductions in dopamine concentration, receptor density, and transporter availability have also been shown to be most pronounced in these late developing areas such as the prefrontal cortex, which effects executive function [8–10].

The frontal lobes control areas of higher functioning responsible for decision making, attention, multitasking, conceptual priming, speech, and articulation. In normal aging we see the ability to focus on one task at a time is maintained, while the ability to shift attention between tasks efficiently becomes impaired. This increased distractibility, or inability to put processes "on hold" during other tasks, is a phenomenon seen across multiple species, indicating that this change in function is a biologic process as opposed to a disease process [6, 7]. Normal aging also selectively impairs certain language abilities including speed of speech, word retrieval, and naming. While ventral and dorsal language processing pathways are present at birth, the pathways connecting superior temporal cortex (Wernicke's area) to the inferior frontal cortex (Broca's area) are not present in newborns and develop later in childhood [11–14]. Again, this points to the idea that it is the more complex, later developing neurocognitive domains that are most susceptible to deterioration with aging or "last in, first out."

The temporal lobe is important for memory and spatial navigation, both of which can be impaired in normal aging. Hippocampal volume has been shown to have annual atrophy rates of up to 2 % in normal adults over the age of 40 [8]. Corresponding decline in spatial navigation was shown to be apparent after age 60 and further accelerated after age 70 [15]. Allocentric navigation is a "world-centered" processing of spatial information requiring individuals to rely on a spatial map using distant landmarks and has been shown to be dependent on medial temporal lobe structures, especially the hippocampus, and is impaired in healthy older adults. In contrast, egocentric navigation is a "body-centered" processing of spatial navigation in which distance and directions from an individual's body position are used for navigation. Egocentric navigation is parietal lobe dependent and was shown not to be affected in older adults [16]. This may result in healthy older adults avoiding new environments and becoming restricted to familiar places due to impairment in allocentric navigation. As with navigation, there are different types of memory that functionally differ with the aging hippocampus. Episodic memory, which is a conscious recollection of a person's experienced events, declines most with age. Semantic memory, which are facts, meanings, concepts, and rote knowledge, shows little age-related decline, and physical memory, such as guitar playing or knitting, is the least affected with age [17].

In contrast to frontal and temporal lobes, the parietal lobe is relatively preserved in structure and function with normal aging. The parietal lobe is involved in sensory and somatosensory perception, as well as written and verbal language comprehension. White matter disease in the parietal lobes is not found in healthy older adults and has been shown to predict progression to AD in one large cohort of older, community-dwelling adults, independent of hippocampal volume. In fact, the parietal lobe is where we see the earliest deposition of amyloid plaque pathology and APOE-ε4, the strongest genetic risk factor for late-onset AD [18].

The motor cortex and cerebellum both show physiologic changes with normal aging that are linked to motor, gait, and balance impairment. Muscle strength decreases at a rate of 3 % per year after the age of 70. In conjunction with this decline in muscle strength, adults older than 65 exhibit a 43 % volumetric reduction in the premotor cortex neuron cell body size and have lower glutamate concentrations in motor cortex compared to younger adults [19]. While the number of neurons is stable in numerous cerebral areas, the cerebellum displays a significant loss of neurons with age. Between the ages of 40 and 90, we see an evenly distributed loss of 30–40 % of Purkinje cells over time. Atrophy in these motor and cerebellar areas is associated with reduced motor abilities in aging including coordination difficulty, increased variability of movement, decreased processing and response times, and decreased gait speed [20–23].

What Works to Promote Healthy Brain Aging

Exercise

Exercise has been shown in many studies to maintain or even improve cognitive function. In subjects with subjective memory complaints or MCI, a moderate intensity exercise program improved cognitive scores, and several randomized studies of strength training showed improved executive function, particularly in women [24–27]. Importantly, being active during nonwork time at midlife has been shown to reduce the risk of cognitive decline later in life, so patients should be encouraged to be active at every age [28]. A systematic review of tai chi and cognitive function showed that people with normal cognition had improved executive function and those with cognitive impairment had improved global cognition (as measured by mini-mental status exam). These results held true even when there was an active comparator (such as walking). Risks of tai chi were extremely low, even in somewhat fragile populations. Effects of tai chi are thought to be due to several elements—it is moderately aerobic (similar to brisk walking); it improves agility and mobility; it involves learning and memorization; it includes training in sustained attentional focus, shifting, and multitasking; it is meditative and relaxing; and the social support of classes may enhance cognitive function [29].

Diet

The Mediterranean diet has been shown in randomized controlled trials to improve cardiovascular health, and more recently, this evidence has extended to cognitive health as well. In a cognitively healthy group of Spanish subjects with a mean age of 66, supplementing diet with olive oil or nuts improved auditory verbal learning and executive function compared to controls who were simply given a recommendation to reduce fat in their diet [30]. Epidemiologic data strongly supports the benefits of the Mediterranean diet. Two separate systematic reviews published in 2013 and 2014 found that greater adherence (top tertile compared to bottom tertile of adherence) to a Mediterranean diet reduced risk of developing Alzheimer's disease by 33–40 % and reduced risk of MCI by 27 %. An 11 % reduction in risk of MCI converting to Alzheimer's disease was observed for each unit increase (scale of 1–9) in the Mediterranean diet score [31, 32]. The benefits from the Mediterranean diet have been postulated to be attributable to its reduced risk of coronary disease, hypertension, diabetes, dyslipidemia, and metabolic syndrome, all of which are considered risk factors for cognitive impairment [33–36]. The Mediterranean diet may also reduce C-reactive protein, which has been associated with cognitive decline [37, 38]. Two cohort studies (from the Memory and Aging Project and Cache County, Utah) published in 2014 corroborate the value of the Mediterranean diet to reduce risk of cognitive decline and add evidence to support the value of the Dietary Approaches to Stop Hypertension (DASH) diet in reducing the risk of cognitive decline [39, 40]. Together, these studies lend ample evidence to support close adherence to the Mediterranean diet, and possibly the DASH diet, to reduce the risk of cognitive decline.

Cognitive Training/Stimulation

The largest randomized controlled trial on cognitive training (the Advanced Cognitive Training for Independent and Vital Elderly, or ACTIVE trial, 2832 participants) had four training groups—memory, reasoning, speed of processing, and a no-contact control group. Subjects participated in cognitive training for 10–14 weeks, and in over 10 years of follow-up, the results show cognitive training slows cognitive and functional decline, with the speed of processing group having the biggest overall impact on health status [41, 42]. Other smaller studies show more mixed effects [43], and overall, the improvement is fairly modest, but cognitive training options are widely available via cognitive therapy and online venues and can be easily incorporated into the daily regimen of brain protection activities.

Creativity

A randomized controlled trial of 166 healthy older adults engaging in creative activity (chorale group) reduced doctor visits, medication use, and falls and led to better morale, less loneliness, and higher levels of activity [44]. A smaller study of community-dwelling older adults randomized to a theater group, visual art group, or a control group found that the theater group showed improvement in recall and problem solving [45]. Pursuit of creative endeavors also encourages social engagement, which has also been shown to preserve memory function in large observational trials [46, 47]. And one study enrolled 119 subjects into groups of exercise plus musical accompaniment, exercise alone, or a control group and found that the group who received exercise and music had more positive effects on cognition than either of the other groups [48]. So dancing may be better than walking, and learning a new musical instrument may be better than doing computer-based cognitive training.

Sleep

Sleep disturbance may also be linked to dementia and cognitive decline in older adults. Excess beta-amyloid builds up in the interstitial spaces of the brain due to overproduction, reduced clearance, or both. The concentration of beta-amyloid in interstitial and cerebrospinal fluid varies, depending on whether a person is asleep or awake: beta-amyloid concentration dips during sleep and peaks during consciousness. This suggests that sleep-wake patterns affect fluctuations in beta-amyloid concentration. Rodent studies recently found that sleep changes the cellular structure of the brain and plays a critical role in beta-amyloid clearance. This suggests that sleep helps the brain dispose of metabolic waste that accumulates while awake. If similar results are found in humans, sleep length and quality could be modifiable risk factors, and interventions to improve sleep or maintain healthy sleep might help prevent or slow AD [49].

Counseling Patients for Healthy Brain Aging

In the IOM report mentioned at the beginning of this chapter, clinicians are encouraged to:

1. "Identify risk factors for cognitive decline and recommend measures to minimize risk and review patient medications, paying attention to medications known to have an impact on cognition"
2. "Provide patients and families with information on cognitive aging (as distinct from dementia) and actions that they can take to maintain cognitive health and prevent cognitive decline"
3. "Encourage individuals and family members to discuss their concerns and questions regarding cognitive health" [3]

Counseling patients about lifestyle factors that may help reduce risk of cognitive decline, notably those discussed above, should be part of routine care of older adults, as should regular medication review and reduction when possible. In addition, recognizing "normal or not" can be critical to counseling patients about cognitive changes they are noticing. Some simple guidelines for recognizing "normal or not" are:

- Some degree of white matter atrophy is normal with aging.
- Atrophy in AD follows a specific pattern *not* seen in normal aging.
- Impairments in the following functions (without impacting ADLs) can be expected in *normal* aging:
  - Multitasking
  - Slowed speech
  - Word retrieval

  - Naming
  - Allocentric spatial navigation
  - Episodic memory
  - Motor coordination
  - Motor response time
  - Balance and gait
- Impairments in these functions are *not* normal with aging and are associated with dementia:
  - Visual-motor tasks
  - Egocentric spatial navigation
  - Semantic memory
  - Physical memory
  - Sensory/somatosensory perception
  - Written/spoken language comprehension

Clinicians are often hesitant to open the "black box" of cognitive concerns, but research shows that most older people care about their cognitive health [50], and in one screening study, patients reported they "have no concerns or that they were pleased to have [their] memory evaluated." [51] The Alzheimer's Association and other patient advocacy groups recommend early diagnosis and care planning to ensure optimal quality of care for patients with dementia. While no studies have determined the best way to deliver a diagnosis or discuss difficult future decisions such as retiring from driving or moving to a memory care facility, we encourage the following steps (modeled after the SPIKES tool) [52, 53]:

1. **S—SETTING UP the interview**. Be sure the right people are in the room. This usually includes the spouse and any adult children or friends who are (or could become) engaged in caregiving and may need to happen at a separate appointment from the cognitive evaluation so that important family members can be present.
2. **P—Assessing the patient's PERCEPTION**. Start by asking the patient how they think their memory has been doing or if they have noticed any trouble with complex tasks such as driving. If the patient allows, ask family members for their perceptions. Ask open-ended questions, and ask how much the patient and family want to know about what to expect in the future.
3. **I—Obtaining the patient's INVITATION**. Ask the patient if you may describe what you found during your cognitive evaluation. If you are disclosing a diagnosis of mild cognitive impairment or dementia, be as specific as you can be about the diagnosis (e.g., Alzheimer's versus Lewy body disease) and stop after you say it to let it sink in. Think of this in a similar way to disclosing a diagnosis of cancer.
4. **K—Giving KNOWLEDGE and information to the patient**. Provide as many details as the patient wants to hear about symptoms, prognosis, and what to expect down the road (behavioral symptoms, eventual loss of ability to swallow and walk, etc.). Check frequently for understanding, and frame the discussion in

light of the patient's goals for their life. Often this part of the conversation takes multiple visits over time to prevent the patient and family from becoming overwhelmed.

5. **E—Addressing the patient's EMOTIONS with empathic responses**. Articulate emotions you are recognizing ("I can tell this is a scary diagnosis for you"), and empathize with the seriousness of the diagnosis. Express support for the patient and family and ongoing care and communication at every stage of the disease.

6. **S—STRATEGY and SUMMARY**. Review strategies to maintain the best possible quality of life, including all of the preventive strategies described above. Solicit patient and family feedback about next steps and provide resources such as the Alzheimer's Association (alz.org). Schedule a follow-up appointment soon to address further questions and concerns.

Summary

Alzheimer's disease and related dementias currently cannot be completely prevented, but it has been said that delaying onset even just 5 years could reduce the cost to society by 50 %. Healthy lifestyle could help maintain cognitive function and is valuable for people of all ages. Exercise, healthy diet, cognitive stimulation, creative engagement, and healthy sleep show promise in reducing the risk of cognitive decline, yet few older adults practice these behaviors on a regular basis. Counseling and resource provision to enhance uptake of healthy cognitive behaviors could have a substantial impact on patients, family members, caregivers, and our entire society.

Key Points

1. While drugs and supplements have disappointed in preventing cognitive decline, lifestyle modification, such as healthy diet, exercise, creativity, cognitive stimulation, and good sleep, may be helpful.

2. The Mediterranean diet has been shown in randomized controlled trials to improve cardiovascular health, and more recently, this evidence has extended to cognitive health as well.

3. Being active during nonwork time at midlife has been shown to reduce the risk of cognitive decline later in life, so patients should be encouraged to be active at every age.

4. A systematic review of tai chi and cognitive function showed that people with normal cognition had improved executive function and those with cognitive impairment had improved global cognition.

5. Cognitive training slows cognitive and functional decline, with the speed of processing group having the biggest overall impact on health status.

6. Pursuit of creative endeavors encourages social engagement, which has also been shown to preserve memory function in large.

7. Sleep length and quality could be modifiable risk factors, and interventions to improve sleep or maintain healthy sleep might help prevent or slow cognitive loss.
8. While no studies have determined the best way to deliver a diagnosis of memory loss, steps (modeled after the SPIKES tool) can be taken to guide the discussion.

References

1. Cheng G, Huang C, Deng H, Wang H. Diabetes as a risk factor for dementia and mild cognitive impairment: a meta-analysis of longitudinal studies. Intern Med J. 2012;42(5):484–91.
2. Alzheimer's Association. 2015 Alzheimer's disease facts and figures. Alzheimers Dement. 2015;11(3)332.
3. IOM (Institute of Medicine). 2015. Cognitive aging: Progress in understanding and opportunities for action. Washington, DC: The National Academies Press.
4. Guttmann CR, Jolesz FA, Kikinis R, Killiany RJ, Moss MB, Sandor T, et al. White matter changes with normal aging. Neurology. 1998;50(4):972–8.
5. Buckner RL. Memory and executive function in aging and AD: multiple factors that cause decline and reserve factors that compensate. Neuron. 2004;44(1):195–208.
6. Cabeza R, Dennis NA. Frontal lobes and aging: deterioration and compensation. In: Stuss DT, Knight RT, editors. Principles of frontal lobe function. 2nd ed. New York: Oxford University Press; 2013.
7. Bloom FE, Beal MF, Kupfer DJ, editors. The Dana guide to brain health: a practical family reference from medical experts. New York: Dana Press; 2006.
8. Fjell AM, McEvoy L, Holland D, Dale AM, Walhovd KB, Alzheimer's Disease Neuroimaging Initiative. What is normal in normal aging? Effects of aging, amyloid and Alzheimer's disease on the cerebral cortex and the hippocampus. Prog Neurobiol. 2014;117:20–40.
9. Vanguilder HD, Freeman WM. The hippocampal neuroproteome with aging and cognitive decline: past progress and future directions. Front Aging Neurosci. 2011;3:8.
10. Khan ZU, Martin-Montanez E, Navarro-Lobato I, Muly EC. Memory deficits in aging and neurological diseases. Prog Mol Biol Transl Sci. 2014;122:1–29.
11. Bidelman GM, Villafuerte JW, Moreno S, Alain C. Age-related changes in the subcortical-cortical encoding and categorical perception of speech. Neurobiol Aging. 2014;35(11):2526–40.
12. McDowd J, Hoffman L, Rozek E, Lyons KE, Pahwa R, Burns J, et al. Understanding verbal fluency in healthy aging, Alzheimer's disease, and Parkinson's disease. Neuropsychology. 2011;25(2):210–25.
13. Shafto MA, Tyler LK. Language in the aging brain: the network dynamics of cognitive decline and preservation. Science. 2014;346(6209):583–7.
14. Yang Y, Dai B, Howell P, Wang X, Li K, Lu C. White and grey matter changes in the language network during healthy aging. PLoS One. 2014;9(9):e108077.
15. Barrash J. A historical review of topographical disorientation and its neuroanatomical correlates. J Clin Exp Neuropsychol. 1998;20(6):807–27.
16. Gazova I, Laczo J, Rubinova E, Mokrisova I, Hyncicova E, Andel R, et al. Spatial navigation in young versus older adults. Front Aging Neurosci. 2013;5:94.
17. Park DC, Smith AD, Lautenschlager G, Earles JL, Frieske D, Zwahr M, et al. Mediators of long-term memory performance across the life span. Psychol Aging. 1996;11(4):621–37.
18. Brickman AM, Zahodne LB, Guzman VA, Narkhede A, Meier IB, Griffith EY, et al. Reconsidering harbingers of dementia: progression of parietal lobe white matter hyperintensities predicts Alzheimer's disease incidence. Neurobiol Aging. 2015;36(1):27–32.

19. Boisgontier MP. Motor aging results from cerebellar neuron death. Trends Neurosci. 2015;38(3):127–8.
20. Bernard JA, Seidler RD. Moving forward: age effects on the cerebellum underlie cognitive and motor declines. Neurosci Biobehav Rev. 2014;42:193–207.
21. Clark BC, Taylor JL. Age-related changes in motor cortical properties and voluntary activation of skeletal muscle. Curr Aging Sci. 2011;4(3):192–9.
22. Nadkarni NK, Nunley KA, Aizenstein H, Harris TB, Yaffe K, Satterfield S, et al. Association between cerebellar gray matter volumes, gait speed, and information-processing ability in older adults enrolled in the Health ABC study. J Gerontol A Biol Sci Med Sci. 2014;69(8):996–1003.
23. Seidler RD, Bernard JA, Burutolu TB, Fling BW, Gordon MT, Gwin JT, et al. Motor control and aging: links to age-related brain structural, functional, and biochemical effects. Neurosci Biobehav Rev. 2010;34(5):721–33.
24. Porto FH, Coutinho AM, Pinto AL, Gualano B, Duran FL, Prando S, et al. Effects of aerobic training on cognition and brain glucose metabolism in subjects with mild cognitive impairment. J Alzheimers Dis. 2015;46:747–60.
25. Liu-Ambrose T, Nagamatsu LS, Graf P, Beattie BL, Ashe MC, Handy TC. Resistance training and executive functions: a 12-month randomized controlled trial. Arch Intern Med. 2010;170(2):170–8.
26. Lautenschlager NT, Cox KL, Flicker L, Foster JK, van Bockxmeer FM, Xiao J, et al. Effect of physical activity on cognitive function in older adults at risk for Alzheimer disease: a randomized trial. JAMA. 2008;300(9):1027–37.
27. Baker LD, Frank LL, Foster-Schubert K, Green PS, Wilkinson CW, McTiernan A, et al. Effects of aerobic exercise on mild cognitive impairment: a controlled trial. Arch Neurol. 2010;67(1):71–9.
28. Rovio S, Kareholt I, Helkala EL, Viitanen M, Winblad B, Tuomilehto J, et al. Leisure-time physical activity at midlife and the risk of dementia and Alzheimer's disease. Lancet Neurol. 2005;4(11):705–11.
29. Wayne PM, Walsh JN, Taylor-Piliae RE, Wells RE, Papp KV, Donovan NJ, et al. Effect of tai chi on cognitive performance in older adults: systematic review and meta-analysis. J Am Geriatr Soc. 2014;62(1):25–39.
30. Valls-Pedret C, Sala-Vila A, Serra-Mir M, Corella D, de la Torre R, Martinez-Gonzalez MA, et al. Mediterranean diet and age-related cognitive decline: a randomized clinical trial. JAMA Intern Med. 2015;175:1094–103.
31. Lourida I, Soni M, Thompson-Coon J, Purandare N, Lang IA, Ukoumunne OC, et al. Mediterranean diet, cognitive function, and dementia: a systematic review. Epidemiology. 2013;24(4):479–89.
32. Singh B, Parsaik AK, Mielke MM, Erwin PJ, Knopman DS, Petersen RC, et al. Association of Mediterranean diet with mild cognitive impairment and Alzheimer's disease: a systematic review and meta-analysis. J Alzheimers Dis. 2014;39(2):271–82.
33. Martinez-Gonzalez MA, de la Fuente-Arrillaga C, Nunez-Cordoba JM, Basterra-Gortari FJ, Beunza JJ, Vazquez Z, et al. Adherence to Mediterranean diet and risk of developing diabetes: prospective cohort study. BMJ. 2008;336(7657):1348–51.
34. Stampfer MJ, Hu FB, Manson JE, Rimm EB, Willett WC. Primary prevention of coronary heart disease in women through diet and lifestyle. N Engl J Med. 2000;343(1):16–22.
35. Panagiotakos DB, Pitsavos CH, Chrysohoou C, Skoumas J, Papadimitriou L, Stefanadis C, et al. Status and management of hypertension in Greece: role of the adoption of a Mediterranean diet: the Attica study. J Hypertens. 2003;21(8):1483–9.
36. Esposito K, Ciotola M, Giugliano D. Mediterranean diet and the metabolic syndrome. Mol Nutr Food Res. 2007;51(10):1268–74.
37. Kuo HK, Yen CJ, Chang CH, Kuo CK, Chen JH, Sorond F. Relation of C-reactive protein to stroke, cognitive disorders, and depression in the general population: systematic review and meta-analysis. Lancet Neurol. 2005;4(6):371–80.

38. Chrysohoou C, Panagiotakos DB, Pitsavos C, Das UN, Stefanadis C. Adherence to the Mediterranean diet attenuates inflammation and coagulation process in healthy adults: the ATTICA Study. J Am Coll Cardiol. 2004;44(1):152–8.
39. Tangney CC, Li H, Wang Y, Barnes L, Schneider JA, Bennett DA, et al. Relation of DASH- and Mediterranean-like dietary patterns to cognitive decline in older persons. Neurology. 2014;83(16):1410–6.
40. Wengreen H, Munger RG, Cutler A, Quach A, Bowles A, Corcoran C, et al. Prospective study of Dietary Approaches to Stop Hypertension- and Mediterranean-style dietary patterns and age-related cognitive change: the Cache County Study on Memory, Health and Aging. Am J Clin Nutr. 2013;98(5):1263–71.
41. Ball K, Berch DB, Helmers KF, Jobe JB, Leveck MD, Marsiske M, et al. Effects of cognitive training interventions with older adults: a randomized controlled trial. JAMA. 2002; 288(18):2271–81.
42. Rebok GW, Ball K, Guey LT, Jones RN, Kim HY, King JW, et al. Ten-year effects of the advanced cognitive training for independent and vital elderly cognitive training trial on cognition and everyday functioning in older adults. J Am Geriatr Soc. 2014;62(1):16–24.
43. Papp KV, Walsh SJ, Snyder PJ. Immediate and delayed effects of cognitive interventions in healthy elderly: a review of current literature and future directions. Alzheimers Dement. 2009;5(1):50–60.
44. Cohen GD, Perlstein S, Chapline J, Kelly J, Firth KM, Simmens S. The impact of professionally conducted cultural programs on the physical health, mental health, and social functioning of older adults. Gerontologist. 2006;46(6):726–34.
45. Noice H, Noice T, Staines G. A short-term intervention to enhance cognitive and affective functioning in older adults. J Aging Health. 2004;16(4):562–85.
46. Ertel KA, Glymour MM, Berkman LF. Effects of social integration on preserving memory function in a nationally representative US elderly population. Am J Public Health. 2008;98(7):1215–20.
47. James BD, Wilson RS, Barnes LL, Bennett DA. Late-life social activity and cognitive decline in old age. J Int Neuropsychol Soc. 2011;17(6):998–1005.
48. Satoh M, Ogawa J, Tokita T, Nakaguchi N, Nakao K, Kida H, et al. The effects of physical exercise with music on cognitive function of elderly people: Mihama-Kiho project. PLoS One. 2014;9(4):e95230.
49. Ju YE, McLeland JS, Toedebusch CD, Xiong C, Fagan AM, Duntley SP, et al. Sleep quality and preclinical Alzheimer disease. JAMA Neurol. 2013;70(5):587–93.
50. 2012 member opinion survey issue spotlight: interests & concerns. 2013. http://www.aarp.org/politics-society/advocacy/info-01-2013/interests-concerns-member-opinion-survey-issue-spotlight.html.
51. Boise L, Eckstrom E, Fagnan L, King A, Goubaud M, Buckley DI, et al. The rural older adult memory (ROAM) study: a practice-based intervention to improve dementia screening and diagnosis. J Am Board Fam Med. 2010;23(4):486–98.
52. Baile WF, Buckman R, Lenzi R, Glober G, Beale EA, Kudelka AP. SPIKES-A six-step protocol for delivering bad news: application to the patient with cancer. Oncologist. 2000;5(4):302–11.
53. Buckman RA. Breaking bad news: the S-P-I-K-E-S strategy. Commun Oncol. 2005;2:138–42.

Targeting Enhanced Services Toward High-Cost, High-Need Medicare Patients

2

Melissa Dattalo, Stephanie Nothelle, and Elizabeth N. Chapman

Theresa is a 65-year-old woman with type 2 diabetes on insulin complicated by neuropathy and nephropathy, congestive heart failure, hypertension, dyslipidemia, stage III chronic kidney disease, obstructive sleep apnea, and depression who was admitted to the hospital with acute decompensation of chronic systolic heart failure. In the week leading up to her current hospitalization, she gained 20 lb and had weeping wounds on her legs with painful edema. Her glycosylated hemoglobin was 13.6 %. She had run out of insulin and missed several doses of her antihypertensive medications. She was new to the hospital system, having recently moved to the area to live with her sister. Theresa was prescribed 12 medications, regularly saw four specialists in her former hometown, and had three hospital admissions for shortness of breath in the past year.

Theresa is an older adult who struggles to manage her multiple chronic conditions (MCC), resulting in frequent hospitalizations and emergency department (ED) visits. The complexity of Theresa's care may remind clinicians across the country of similar patients they see in their hospitals and clinics. These high-cost, high-need patients

M. Dattalo (✉)
Geriatric Research Education and Clinical Center (GRECC), William S. Middleton Memorial VA Hospital, University of Wisconsin-Madison School of Medicine and Public Health, 2500 Overlook Terrace, Madison, WI 53705, USA
e-mail: mdattalo@uwhealth.org

S. Nothelle
Department of Medicine, Johns Hopkins Bayview Medical Center, 5200 Eastern Avenue, Mason F. Lord Center Tower, 2nd floor, Suite 220, Baltimore, MD 21224, USA
e-mail: Snothel1@jhmi.edu

E.N. Chapman
Geriatric Research Education and Clinical Center (GRECC), University of Wisconsin-Madison School of Medicine and Public Health, 2500 Overlook Terrace, 11G, Madison, WI 53705, USA
e-mail: enchapman@medicine.wisc.edu

© Springer International Publishing Switzerland 2016
L.A. Lindquist (ed.), *New Directions in Geriatric Medicine*,
DOI 10.1007/978-3-319-28137-7_2

compose a small proportion of America's population, but account for a majority of our health-care expenditures. Despite these high health-care costs, patients like Theresa do not often receive the optimal health-care services to meet their comprehensive needs. The needs of patients with MCC, functional limitations, and complex social challenges are often mismatched with our fragmented, disease-centered health-care system. This chapter will describe characteristics of high-cost, high-need patients, highlight health-care reforms offering new opportunities to improve their care, and provide an overview of evidence-based models of care that may better meet their comprehensive needs.

Defining High-Cost, High-Need Populations

Although clinicians commonly encounter patients like Theresa, there is little consensus about how to define this vulnerable population and little research exploring the range of variability within this population. Although patients are unlikely to self-identify with existing labels, terms commonly ascribed to this population include "high-utilizers," "super-utilizers," "super-users," and more recently "high-cost, high-need patients" [1]. Definitions are also varied, ranging from qualitative descriptions such as the Centers for Medicare & Medicaid Services (CMS) definition as those who have "complex, unaddressed health issues and a history of frequent encounters with health care providers" [1], to using common statistical practices to define the population as those who are two standard deviations from the norm in their of use of health-care services [2]. Increasingly, the definition has revolved around the issue of cost, as health-care spending nationally continues to soar and hospital utilization accounts for the majority of health-care costs.

Whether words or numbers are used to describe characteristics of this population, individuals identified through these methods are both medically and socially complex. The Agency for Healthcare Research and Quality (AHRQ) defines "complexity" as the magnitude of mismatch between a patient's needs and the services available to him/her in the health-care system and community [3]. This definition may capture the underlying systemic causes of frequent hospitalizations for individuals with complex health needs. On one hand, defining "high-utilizing" individuals based on consumption of health-care resources alone discounts the unmet needs of individuals. Conversely, while individual needs vary, focusing solely on individual needs fails to recognize the system-level challenges and opportunities that these individuals reveal. Thus, we will use the term "high-cost, high-need patients" for the duration of this chapter to emphasize the mismatch between complex individual needs and traditional health-care system resources for this patient population.

Disproportionate Health-Care Costs

The concept that a small proportion of the population can account for a large amount of health-care costs [4, 5] has been receiving increased attention as health-care reform efforts target the "triple aim" of better health, better health care, and better

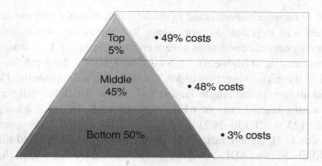

Fig. 2.1 This pyramid represents the distribution of medical expenditures for Americans of all ages, as assessed through the Medical Expenditures Panel Survey in 2002 [8]. The top 5 % of the population accounted for 49 % of health-care expenditures nationally. Conwell LJ, Cohen JW. Characteristics of Persons with High Medical Expenditures in the U.S. Civilian Noninstitutionalized Population, 2002. Rockville, MD: Agency for Healthcare Research and Quality, 2005

value [6]. Across all age groups, 5 % of the population accounts for almost 50 % of annual health-care expenditures (Fig. 2.1), with the top 1 % accounting for 22 % of annual health-care expenditures [7, 8]. One may expect such a skewed distribution when a large portion of healthy individuals are using little to no health-care services, but this distribution also holds true within the Medicare population, where 2/3 of beneficiaries are managing MCC [9]. Within the Medicare fee-for-service program, the top 5 % of beneficiaries account for 39 % of total Medicare spending, and 25 % of beneficiaries account for 82 % of all spending [10].

As the number of chronic conditions rises, so does health-care utilization. High-cost, high-need patients within the Medicare population are the highest utilizers of the hospital [11], and it is through hospital admissions that most costs are accrued. The 14 % of Medicare beneficiaries with six or more chronic conditions account for almost half of all Medicare spending and 70 % of hospital readmissions [9]. Outside of the hospital, those with MCC also utilize home health services more frequently, visit physician's offices more often, and have more ED visits.

Complex Medical Needs

Increasing numbers of chronic conditions are closely associated with increasing health-care costs. Of the top 5 % of Medicare spenders, 93 % have three or more chronic conditions [12]. Certain chronic conditions, such as chronic kidney disease, congestive heart failure, chronic lung disease, anxiety or depression, and cancer, are well-established risk factors for hospital readmission [10, 13–15]. For individuals over the age of 50, depression and cognitive impairment are independent and synergistic risk factors for hospitalization for ambulatory care sensitive conditions [16].

Having MCC alone is not sufficient to explain patterns of frequent hospitalizations. In 2010, almost two out of every five Medicare beneficiaries with six or more chronic conditions were not admitted to the hospital, roughly half did not use post-acute care, and well over half did not engage in home health services despite their MCC [9]. Having chronic conditions severe enough to impact daily function may be a critical characteristic of high-cost, high-need patients. Of the top 5 % of Medicare spenders, 61 % have a combination of MCC and functional limitations [12]. Having a hospital admission is the single largest risk factor for developing a functional impairment with a hazard ratio of 61.8 (95 % CI 49.0–78.0) for a hospitalization alone and 223 (95 % CI 138–362) for a hospitalization with a subsequent nursing home admission [17]. Beneficiaries who have chronic conditions and limitations in activities of daily living (ADLs) average twice the cost of those with three chronic conditions without functional limitations [12].

Patients with MCC often incur high treatment burdens in a health-care system designed to optimize the care of individual diseases in isolation of each other [18, 19]. Guidelines and recommendations for one chronic condition often conflict with that of another, putting patients at risk of therapeutic competition and complications [20]. This fragmented, disease-focused system requires health-care consumers to be savvy and to take an active role communicating among specialists and primary physicians. Most older adults (70 %) self-manage their illnesses, and almost 40 % found this management so burdensome and difficult that they did not complete and or delayed completion of recommended health-related tasks [21]. Difficulties with self-management can be compounded by both cognitive impairment and low health literacy as adults over age 65 have the highest proportion of persons who are below basic levels of health literacy [22].

While many high-cost, high-need patients have potential to achieve stable outpatient management of their conditions with greater supports, some do not enter this population until the last year of life with end-stage illnesses. Almost a third of high-cost, high-need patients are those who are in their last year of life [23]. Health-care spending increases toward the end of life [24], with 30 % of costs for a dying Medicare beneficiary in the last year incurred in the last month of life and 25 % of total Medicare expenditures paid toward decedents in their last year of life [25]. Over time, there have been trends toward more frequent hospitalizations in the last 3 months of life and increasing numbers of deaths in intensive care units concurrently with increased use of the Medicare hospice benefits [26–28]. Despite these utilization trends in the last year of life, the total proportion of Medicare spending toward descendants has remained stable at 5 % of total expenditures [23, 28]. While there is some evidence that those enrolled in hospice have less acute care utilization at the end of life [29] and are less likely to die in the acute hospital [27], studies examining cost-savings of hospice services show mixed results [25, 30–32].

Complex Social Needs

Theresa moved in with her sister after leaving an abusive husband in another state. She left with only her purse and a few medication bottles. Since then, she hadn't had the money to refill her prescriptions and had not been able to establish a new primary care doctor. She had Medicare Part A to cover hospital costs, but was worried about the costs of seeing a physician in clinic as she had not enrolled in Medicare part B. She considered enrolling in Medicare Part D for prescription coverage, but found the paperwork overwhelming and the copays too expensive. She had completed high school, but always struggled with reading.

During previous admissions, Theresa's discharge instructions always advised her to weigh herself daily, to check her blood sugar four times daily, and to eat a special "diabetic diet" limited to "two grams of sodium." She didn't own a scale and was not confident in applying the dietary recommendations to her life, particularly now that she was eating meals prepared by her sister. She limited her blood sugar checks to conserve expensive glucometer test strips. She feared the symptoms associated with past hypoglycemic episodes, so often skipped insulin doses rather than risking low blood sugars. Afraid of being judged for not following medical advice, she avoided following up in clinic after hospital stays.

While some disparate utilization can be expected for medically complex patients, difficulty navigating the health-care system and inadequate attention to social determinants of health can compound medical needs and contribute to high hospital utilization patterns [1, 33]. Social and systemic factors associated with high-cost, high-need populations include having low income, belonging to minority populations, having a history of childhood trauma, and having difficulty accessing primary care [10, 15, 34, 35]. Among Medicare beneficiaries specifically, living alone has been a strong predictor of hospital readmission risk in addition to having new or unmet functional needs, lacking self-management skills, having limited education, and having fair to poor satisfaction with one's primary care physician [36, 37].

Personal factors and goals may also contribute to hospital utilization patterns. Desire for aggressive care has been identified as a strong predictor of future utilization as well as the perception of the primary care provider-patient relationship and the quality of care received from the primary provider [38]. Qualitative analyses of interviews with high-cost, high-need patients have highlighted some perceptions these individuals have of their own care. Some patients express that early-life trauma contributes to difficult interactions with health-care providers as adults and that caring relationships with primary care providers are important to their well-being [35]. Patients have also described choices to go directly to the ED when experiencing symptoms are related to poor primary care access or a belief that primary care was ineffective [39].

The complex medical, social, and functional needs of high-cost, high-need patients represent both challenges in our current health-care system and opportunities for improvement. Greater attention to the context of a patient's illness and the resources available to him/her may allow for better customization of services aligned with individual needs.

Hospitalization Risk Prediction Models for Clinicians

Theresa's age, previous hospital admissions in the past year, and her multiple medical conditions prompted referral to the hospital's transitional care program. A social worker assessed her financial challenges and connected her with access to primary care. Her reading level was estimated to be less than eighth grade, so health information was conveyed using the teach-back method, and she received informational handouts intended for those with low literacy. She was provided a pill box for medication management and a scale at no charge. A transitional care nurse practicioner provided a rapid post-discharge follow-up visit to Theresa the day after she left the hospital. The nurse practitioner reconciled her medications, reinforced the teaching regarding diabetes management and heart failure management begun in the hospital, and helped her call her new primary care provider's office to schedule an urgent visit when it was discovered that her morning blood sugar was >400.

For most individuals, the use of medical resources is not static throughout their lives, and the progression to high utilization of health care usually begins when mounting medical and psychosocial needs exceed the ability of the traditional health-care systems to accommodate them. Researchers have begun exploring how to predict which individuals will reach this threshold but overall, risk prediction models have fair to poor performance at prospectively predicting hospital readmissions. Most risk prediction models account for past utilization and medical comorbidities. However, few include markers of illness severity, overall function, or social determinants of health due to the scarcity of these factors in medical documentation [40].

The Probability of Repeated Admissions (P_{ra}) score is one such prediction model. It is a score to estimate frequency of hospital admissions within 4 years calculated from questionnaires that include medical variables, demographic data, current health-care usage, and nonmedical factors like self-rated health and the presence an informal caregiver [41]. Since its publication in 1995, the P_{ra} has been validated in multiple settings, and the pooled results of these applications have shown the score to have high specificity for predicting elderly individuals who will admit frequently. However, its sensitivity for identifying those at high risk for hospital readmission is limited, and it may miss high-risk individuals who lack the specific risk factors explored in the questionnaire [42].

Because survey responses can be poor and those at highest risk for readmissions may be less apt to complete a questionnaire, other models have been sought. The LACE index, calculated using data available in the medical record, can predict unplanned hospital readmissions and mortality in currently hospitalized patients, which could help target interventions for readmission prevention before a cycle of recurrent admissions has begun. The index relies on four key variables: length of admission, acuity of the admission, comorbid conditions, and emergency room usage [43, 44].

Beyond individual socioeconomic risk factors for hospital utilization, recent studies have demonstrated environmental associations between living in resource-poor neighborhoods and being at risk for 30-day hospital readmissions [45]. The Area Deprivation Index is a measure of neighborhood-level socioeconomic disadvantage based on national census data that independently predicts hospital readmission after controlling for patient and hospital characteristics. The University of Wisconsin Health Innovation Program maintains a publically available tool (www.HIPxChange.org/ADI), where clinicians can look up the Area Deprivation Index associated with any individual patient by entering his/her zip code [45].

Health-Care Reform Affecting Inpatient Care

The inpatient setting has become a target for incentives to reduce health-care spending because high-cost, high-need patients generate the bulk of their costs via hospital admissions. As part of the Affordable Care Act (ACA), the Hospital Readmissions Reduction Program penalizes hospitals for higher than national benchmark readmission rates for certain conditions within 30 days of discharge from an index hospital stay, regardless of whether an individual readmission was considered preventable. Hospitals with rates that are higher than average are subject to financial penalties of 3 % of total reimbursement as of 2015. When these percentages are scaled to a national level, they resulted about $280 million in financial penalties during the first year of the program [9]. These financial incentives have led hospitals to focus more on preventing readmissions, leading to investment in some new resources for high-cost, high-need patients.

Hospital-Based Interventions to Reduce 30-Day Hospital Readmissions

After a hospital stay, the transition from hospital to home can be a hazardous time period for vulnerable patients. Interventions to coordinate care as patients transfer from hospital to home can improve patient safety and help hospitals avoid financial penalties. While transitional care interventions vary in scope and intensity, they have consistently yielded reductions in short-term hospital readmissions. The Care Transitions Intervention (CTI) is a successful model of transitional care that can be adapted to many contexts. It consists of four principle activities delivered by a registered nurse serving as a Care Transitions Coach®: (1) improved communication facilitated by a personal health record, (2) medication reconciliation and self-management coaching, (3) patient-scheduled follow-up appointments, and (4) patient knowledge of worsening clinical symptoms and how to respond [46]. CTI has reduced readmissions and lowered costs for community-dwelling adults 65 years and older who had been admitted to the hospital [47]. While the CTI was originally delivered by registered nurses during home visits, an adaptation of the CTI delivered by a nurse case manager over the telephone also demonstrated reductions in readmission rates [48].

In general, multicomponent interventions that support patient capacity for self-care are more successful at reducing 30-day readmissions than single-component interventions without patient or caregiver engagement [49]. Interventions can be classified into three categories: (1) predischarge (patient education, medication reconciliation, comprehensive discharge planning, scheduling follow-up appointments prior to discharge), (2) post-discharge (follow-up telephone calls, patient hotlines, enhanced communication with outpatient providers, timely outpatient follow-up, and post-discharge home visits), and (3) bridging interventions (transition coaches, physician continuity from the inpatient to outpatient setting, and patient-centered discharge instructions) [50]. Hospitals are increasingly assembling readmission review teams, which offer data-driven opportunities to identify frequently admitted outliers. Readmission reviews are most effective when chart reviews are supplemented by patient, caregiver, and provider interviews to better understand the challenges these individuals face in the post-discharge period [51]. Readmission reviews can facilitate the identification of system-level care coordination deficits and offer an opportunity to connect high-cost, high-need patients to enhanced outpatient services.

Health-Care Reform Affecting Outpatient Care

Theresa built a strong relationship with her new primary care provider who worked closely with a social worker and the transitional care team to support her during her return home from the hospital. The clinic nurse called Theresa frequently to review her most recent weights and blood sugar values. Her provider documented these encounters carefully and used the transitional care management (TCM) billing codes to increase her reimbursement for the work.

After completing a 30-day period of outpatient management without returning to the hospital, Theresa's transitional care nurse referred her to a complex case management program affiliated with her primary care clinic. Theresa has been working with her case management team, which includes both a nurse and a social worker, to obtain adequate health-care coverage, find stable housing, seek low-cost legal counsel to help with her divorce from her husband, connect with community-based chronic disease self-management support services, and manage her medical problems with the multiple specialists involved in her care. Her primary care physician works closely with the case management team and is able to seek reimbursement for these care coordination services through Medicare's new chronic care management (CCM) billing code. Theresa has not been admitted to the hospital in 3 months, sees her primary care physician regularly, and reports an improved outlook on her health.

In addition to establishing financial penalties to hospitals with higher than expected readmission rates, the ACA has changed health-care financing to incentivize a wide array of health-care reform in the outpatient setting. Accountable Care Organizations (ACOs) allow for shared savings between health-care organizations and Medicare. The shared savings provide an incentive for organizations to invest in new health-care delivery models outside the scope of traditional fee-for-service health-care services. The ACO model allows health-care organizations to remedy many of the systemic ills that lead to ineffective care, decreasing acute care utilization and generating savings [52].

In addition to ACOs, several recent health-care reforms provide opportunities to enhance services for high-cost, high-need patients and shift some of their health-care utilization from inpatient to outpatient settings. Since over three million older adults with functional impairments are homebound [53], Medicare is evaluating the effectiveness of home-based primary care through the Independence at Home Demonstration Project. High-risk patients are selected for Independence at Home services who have ≥2 chronic conditions, who need assistance with ≥2 ADLs, and who have had a hospital admission with subacute rehabilitation or home health post-acute care in the year prior to enrollment [54]. Preliminary results show that the Independence at Home Demonstration Project improved quality of care while saving Medicare $25 million dollars, or an average of $3070 per participating beneficiary [55]. Even practices funded by traditional fee-for-service reimbursement structures can begin to enhance outpatient services through new Medicare billing codes. TCM and CCM billing codes offer new opportunities for adoption of evidence-based care coordination services. Medicare will also begin to reimburse physicians for goals of care conversations and end-of-life counseling in 2016 [56].

New Incentives for Care Coordination

While hospitals can be penalized for failing to prevent readmissions, outpatient clinics can earn additional revenue for coordinating care for vulnerable patients. The TCM codes 99495 and 99496 allow a physician or nonphysician practitioner to receive a higher rate of reimbursement for coordinating the care of a beneficiary discharging from multiple settings, including inpatient or observation hospital stays, skilled nursing facilities, long-term acute care facilities, rehabilitation hospitals, or community mental health center partial hospitalization programs (Table 2.1) [57]. Transitional care services must include communication with a patient or caregiver within 2 days of discharge, medication reconciliation, coordination with both hospital and community services, and a face-to-face post-discharge visit within either a 7-day period (99495) or 14-day period (99496) after discharge. Meeting the requirements to bill for these codes can be challenging, but when done correctly, this billing code generates about 15 % more revenue than a moderate or high acuity office visit would generate alone [57].

In January 2015, Medicare began offering incentives for care management services with the CCM billing code 99490. Care management encompasses a broad range of activities that assist high-risk patients and their families in managing medical and psychosocial challenges with the ultimate goals of improving care quality and reducing care costs [58]. Most high-quality research studies evaluating care management interventions have demonstrated improved quality of care and quality of life outcomes, but utilization outcomes have been mixed [58, 59]. Care management programs that have achieved the dual aims of higher quality and reduced costs share several common characteristics: (1) selecting patients at high risk for hospitalization, yet without such advanced illness such that hospice services would be more beneficial, (2) in-person encounters, including home visits, (3) specially trained care

Table 2.1 Comparison of key requirements for Medicare's transitional care management (TCM) and chronic care management (CCM) fee-for-service billing codes

	Transitional care management (TCM) [57]	Chronic care management (CCM) [60, 63]
Patients eligible for services	Patients discharged home from hospitals or facilities	Patients with ≥2 chronic conditions that place the patient at risk of death, acute exacerbation, or functional decline
Practitioners eligible to bill for services	Physicians, advanced practice nurses, physician assistants, clinical nurse specialists, certified nurse midwives	Physicians, advanced practice nurses, physician assistants, clinical nurse specialists, certified nurse midwives
Patient consent required	None	Written consent maintained in medical record
Non-face-to-face requirement	Communication with patient or caregiver within 2 business days of discharge, care management services	≥20 min/month of care coordination performed or supervised by the practitioner
Additional requirements	Medication reconciliation by date of face-to-face visit	Certified EHR, electronic care plan, 24/7 access, transitional care, care coordination
Reimbursement	2.11 (99495) or 3.05 (99496) relative value units (RVUs)	$40.39 per patient per month in 2015

managers with low caseloads, (4) multidisciplinary teams that involve physicians, especially when care managers are co-located in primary care practices, (5) engagement of informal caregivers, and (6) coaching patients and families in self-management skills [58].

The Medicare CCM billing code 99490 specifies the patients eligible for care management services and provides a structure for their delivery. Medicare beneficiaries are eligible for CCM services if they have ≥2 chronic conditions that place them at significant risk of death, acute exacerbation/decompensation, or functional decline [60, 61]. If such beneficiaries provide written consent to receive CCM services, qualifying practices may bill for at least 20 min of non-face-to-face care coordination activities per month per beneficiary. Only one provider may bill this code per patient per month and it may not be used in conjunction with the TCM codes. These services are reimbursed at $40.39 per patient per month, so could generate almost $100,000 additional revenue for 200 enrolled patients [62, 63]. Depending on the number of patients enrolled, this reimbursement mechanism may provide enough revenue for an average primary care practice to hire a nurse case manager who can be co-located within the practice. In order to bill Medicare for CCM, a practice must offer seven CCM components [60]. The practice itself must offer continuous access to the care team and electronic medical records after-hours, continuity with a designated provider, and multiple avenues of communication (e.g., telephone, web portals) [60, 63]. Clinicians must generate comprehensive care plans that address patients' medical, cognitive, functional, and psychosocial needs in the context of their environments, support networks, and goals of care [60].

Clinicians must also manage patients' chronic conditions, manage care transitions, and coordinate with home- and community-based services to support psychosocial and functional needs [60, 63]. Geriatricians at the University of California, San Francisco developed a four-step pathway for primary care physicians to meet the CCM comprehensive care plan requirement, called the CARES tool. The four steps include: (1) determine the likelihood of care and coordination needs, (2) establish goals of care, (3) assess medical, functional, psychosocial, and environmental care needs, and (4) match resources to needs [60].

Hot Spotting for High-Cost, High-Need Patients

A key component to the ACO model is the concept of "population health management" or panel management. Population health can be defined as "the health outcomes of a group of individuals, including the distribution of such outcomes within the group" [64]. Whether the population of interest is as small as a primary care panel or as large as a geographic county, population-level data allows individuals within the population to be stratified by the complexity of their needs helping to match services to needs. A major area of research interest is better understanding how to match the optimal health-care innovations with the specific populations who are most likely to benefit [65].

Models of care that target the outliers with the highest utilization rates of inpatient services are often called "hot spotting." The use of this term within health care originated from the work of Jeffrey Brenner, who created population health data tracking systems and developed the Camden Coalition of Healthcare Providers to reach beyond clinic walls into the community for low-income patients in Camden, NJ [66]. By geocoding patients' addresses, eight buildings within the city plus the homeless population were identified to account for $12.5 million in health-care expenditures [66]. Geocoding of health-care costs and isolating "hot spots" can help identify social and environmental influences on health and hospital utilization most relevant to local populations.

The Camden Coalition of Healthcare Providers serves high-cost, high-need patients of all ages and bases its care model on the principle that understanding outliers provides information about failures of health-care and community systems. The organization uses data to identify and engage patients who inform system redesign [67]. The organization has developed a cross-site learning collaborative for others interested in "hot spotting" [68] and offers annual mini-grants to teams of health professional students interested in working with high-cost, high-need patients in their own communities [69]. The Association of American Medical Colleges (AAMC) has published a 10-step "Guide to Hot Spotting" for medical students. It focuses on having trainees identify and work with individual patients with patterns of frequent utilization longitudinally through a number of experiences including visiting a patient at home to get to know them as a person, accompanying them to medical visits, and identifying and helping the patient work on factors contributing to utilization (www.aamc.org/hotspotter) [70]. Any health-care provider or trainee can follow the AAMC guide to hot spotting with institutional support. The ultimate goal of the trainee "hot spotting" experience is to use lessons learned from the in-depth case analysis to engage administrators and educators in systems change.

Comprehensive Primary Care for Patients with Multiple Chronic Conditions (MCC)

While geriatric models of care have not traditionally been studied only in high-cost, high-need populations, they have generally been studied in populations of older adults with MCC and/or functional deficits. Since it is known that Medicare beneficiaries with both MCC and functional deficits account for more disproportionate health-care costs than those with chronic conditions alone, geriatric models of care may provide important insights into how to care for high-cost, high-need populations [12].

Almost all outpatient geriatric models of care are grounded in the Chronic Care Model, which has informed many interventions that demonstrated improved health outcomes for patients since its conceptualization in 2000 [71]. The Chronic Care Model is a conceptual framework for optimizing health delivery services for individuals living with chronic illnesses. It requires collaboration between health systems and communities to build an infrastructure for support in six areas: self-management support, decision support, delivery system design, clinical information systems, health-care organization, and community resources. This care delivery framework enables health-care systems to offer proactive, team-based care to support patients in becoming both informed of and engaged in their care, facilitating interactions that lead to improved health outcomes [72]. The Patient-Centered Medical Home (PCMH) is a widely disseminated intervention based on principles of the Chronic Care Model. While large-scale studies of PCMH have not demonstrated cost-savings [73], a potential concern about PCMH implementation is that the intervention may have been targeted too broadly rather than focusing on the high-risk patients who had the most potential to benefit [74].

Many foundational components of comprehensive primary care models align with the required activities for Medicare's CCM billing code described above. Multidisciplinary teams provide comprehensive assessments, development and implementation of evidence-based care plans, communication among all specialties and facilities involved in a patient's care, coordination of care transitions, and connection with home- and community-based resources [75]. The Program of All-Inclusive Care for the Elderly (PACE) is the most established and long-standing model for delivering such comprehensive primary care, but requires special financing with monthly capitated payments from Medicare and Medicaid per member per year. PACE provides team-based primary care and community supports specifically for low-income (Medicaid-eligible), nursing home-eligible Medicare beneficiaries who wish to remain living in their community homes. PACE patients have longer survival and lower rates of hospitalizations and emergency room visits than similar patients in traditional care systems [75, 76].

Comprehensive primary care can also be supported in more traditionally structured primary care practices through comanagement models with geriatric multidisciplinary teams. The Geriatric Resources for Assessment and Care of Elders (GRACE) is a home-based care management model where an off-site multidisciplinary geriatric team comanages low-income older adults in conjunction with their previously established primary care providers [77]. An advanced practice nurse and social work team form a mobile unit that communicates among patients in their homes, the multidisciplinary geriatric team, and the primary care provider. GRACE has demonstrated improved quality of care and reductions in hospitalizations and emergency rooms visits for high-risk subgroups of older adults (P_{ra} score ≥ 0.4), but has not demonstrated cost-savings for lower risk populations [78]. In conjunction with new ACO models, GRACE has now been implemented in multiple sites around the country specifically targeting older adults with MCC, socioeconomic stressors, and ≥ 1 functional impairment, consistently demonstrating reductions in hospitalizations and readmissions [79].

Community-Based Programs for Older Adults

Evidence-based interventions that improve outcomes for older adults with MCC have disseminated more rapidly through community-based organizations than they have through the health-care system. About $20 million per year in federal funding from the Older Americans Act supports the dissemination of evidence-based health promotion programs through Area Agencies on Aging and affiliated organizations throughout the country [80].

One example of the greater than 30 community-based programs that meet the National Council on Aging's highest-tier criteria [81] for evidence-based health promotion programs is the Chronic Disease Self-Management Program (CDSMP). The CDSMP is a 6-week workshop, designed by researchers at Stanford University, which promotes generic self-management skills applying to problems of MCC rather than skills that apply to a specific disease. It is led by lay leaders who have chronic conditions themselves and supports behavior change through role modeling and self-mastery [82]. The program has decreased emergency room visits and hospitalizations for its participants in both randomized controlled trials and real-world effectiveness studies [82, 83]. Clinicians can find community organizations licensed to deliver CDSMP workshops in their states by visiting the Stanford School of Medicine Patient Education and Resource Center website [84]. Other evidence-based community workshops address fall prevention, caregiver support, pain management, and disease management.

Summary

There are many inpatient, outpatient, and community-based services that can meet the complex needs of high-cost, high-need Medicare patients. Twenty-first-century health-care reform offers new opportunities to translate evidence-based models of care for complex patients into practice. New care delivery models such as ACOs and home-based primary care can improve quality of care and reduce costs. New incentives, such as hospital readmission penalties and outpatient reimbursement for care coordination, can also help traditional health-care delivery systems to enhance services for high-cost, high-need Medicare patients.

8–10 Take-Home Points

1. High-cost, high-need patients account for disproportionate health-care costs. In the Medicare population, 5 % of fee-for-service beneficiaries account for 39 % of total Medicare spending.
2. Many of the high-cost health-care services are repeated hospitalizations, with hospitalization being recognized as one of the most expensive medical interventions.
3. Medical, social, and functional complexity contributes to frequent hospitalizations. The AHRQ Multiple Chronic Conditions Research Network defines complexity as the magnitude of mismatch between a patient's needs and the services available to him/her in the health-care system and community.
4. Of the top 5 % of Medicare spenders, 93 % have three or more chronic conditions (MCC). 61 % have a combination of MCC and functional limitations.
5. Social and systemic risk factors associated with frequent hospitalization include living alone, low socioeconomic status, non-White race, history of childhood trauma, lack of self-management skills, poor primary care access, and low satisfaction with one's primary care provider.
6. High-cost, high-need patients can benefit from transitional care in the inpatient and outpatient settings. Medicare started reimbursing outpatient providers for transitional care management in 2013.
7. High-cost, high-need patients can benefit from care management. Medicare started reimbursing outpatient providers for chronic care management in 2015.
8. Models of care that target the outliers with the highest utilization rates of inpatient services are often called "hot spotting." Trainees can engage in hot spotting with faculty support, using lessons learned from in-depth case analyses to engage administrators and educators in systems change.
9. Multiple models exist to help assess and meet the needs of patients with multiple chronic conditions. These models emphasize individualized care that addresses both medical and nonmedical needs, using a team-based approach.

References

1. Mann C. Targeting medicaid super-utilizers to decrease costs and improve quality. Baltimore: Centers of Medicare and Medicaid Services; 2013.
2. Jiang H, Weiss A, Barrett M, Sheng M. Characteristics of hospital stays for super-utilizers by payer, 2012. Rockville: Agency for Healthcare Research and Quality; 2015.
3. Grembowski D, Schaefer J, Johnson KE, Fischer H, Moore SL, Tai-Seale M, et al. A conceptual model of the role of complexity in the care of patients with multiple chronic conditions. Med Care. 2014;52 Suppl 3:S7–14.

4. Densen P, Shapiro S, Einhorn M. Concerning high and low utilizers of service in a medical care plan, and the persistence of utilization levels over a three year period. Milbank Q. 1959;37(3):217–50.
5. Gawande A. The hot spotters: can we lower medical costs by giving the neediest patients better care? The New Yorker. 2011.
6. Berwick DM, Nolan TW, Whittington J. The triple aim: care, health, and cost. Health Aff (Millwood). 2008;27(3):759–69.
7. Cohen SB. The concentration of health care expenditures and related expenses for costly medical conditions, Statistical Brief #455. Rockville, Md.: Agency for Healthcare Research and Quality, Jan. 2012.
8. Conwell LJ, Cohen JW. Characteristics of persons with high medical expenditures in the U.S. civilian noninstitutionalized population, 2002. Rockville: Agency for Healthcare Research and Quality; 2005.
9. Chronic Conditions among Medicare Beneficiaries, Chartbook 2012 Edition. Baltimore: Centers for Medicare and Medicaid Services; 2012.
10. Medicare Payment Advisory Commission. Health care spending and the medicare program: a data book. Washington, DC: Medicare Payment Advisory Commission; 2014.
11. Moore B, Levit K, Elixhauser A. Costs for hospital stays in the United States, 2012. Rockville: Agency for Healthcare Research and Quality; 2014.
12. Komisar H, Feder J. Transforming care for Medicare beneficiaries with chronic conditions and long-term care needs: coordinating care across all services. The SCAN Foundation, October 2011; http://www.thescanfoundation.org/sites/default/files/Georgetown_Trnsfrming_Care.pdf. Cited 17 July 2015.
13. Mather JF, Fortunato GJ, Ash JL, Davis MJ, Kumar A. Prediction of pneumonia 30-day readmissions: a single-center attempt to increase model performance. Respir Care. 2014;59(2):199–208.
14. Donze J, Lipsitz S, Bates DW, Schnipper JL. Causes and patterns of readmissions in patients with common comorbidities: retrospective cohort study. BMJ. 2013;347:f7171.
15. Joynt KE, Gawande AA, Orav EJ, Jha AK. Contribution of preventable acute care spending to total spending for high-cost Medicare patients. JAMA. 2013;309(24):2572–8.
16. Davydow D, Zivin K, Katon W, Pontone G, Chwastiak L, Langa K, et al. Neuropsychiatric disorders and potentially preventable hospitalizations in a prospective cohort study of older Americans. J Gen Intern Med. 2014;29(10):1362–71.
17. Gill TM. Disentangling the disabling process: insights from the precipitating events project. Gerontologist. 2014;54(4):533–49.
18. Boyd CM, Darer J, Boult C, Fried LP, Boult L, Wu AW. Clinical practice guidelines and quality of care for older patients with multiple comorbid diseases: implications for pay for performance. JAMA. 2005;294(6):716–24.
19. Tinetti ME, Fried TR, Boyd CM. Designing health care for the most common chronic condition--multimorbidity. JAMA. 2012;307(23):2493–4.
20. Lorgunpai SJ, Grammas M, Lee DSH, McAvay G, Charpentier P, Tinetti ME. Potential therapeutic competition in community-living older adults in the U.S.: use of medications that may adversely affect a coexisting condition. PLoS One. 2014;9(2):e89447.
21. Wolff J, Boyd C. Erratum to: a look at person- and family-centered care among older adults: results from a national survey. J Gen Intern Med. 2015;30(10):1567.
22. Mark Kutner EG, Ying Jin, Christine Paulsen, Sheida White. The health literacy of America's adults: Results from the 2003 National Assessment of Adult Literacy (NCES 2006-483). U.S. Department of Education. Washington, DC: National Center for Education Statistics; Sept 2006. https://nces.ed.gov/pubs2006/2006483_1.pdf.
23. Lubitz JD, Riley GF. Trends in medicare payments in the last year of life. N Engl J Med. 1993;328(15):1092–6.
24. Hogan C, Lunney J, Gabel J, Lynn J. Medicare beneficiaries' costs of care in the last year of life. Health Aff (Millwood). 2001;20(4):188–95.

25. Emanuel EJ, Ash A, Yu W, Gazelle G, Levinsky NG, Saynina O, et al. Managed care, hospice use, site of death, and medical expenditures in the last year of life. Arch Intern Med. 2002;162(15):1722–8.
26. Barnato AE, McClellan MB, Kagay CR, Garber AM. Trends in inpatient treatment intensity among Medicare beneficiaries at the end of life. Health Serv Res. 2004;39(2):363–75.
27. Teno JM, Gozalo PL, Bynum JW, et al. Change in end-of-life care for medicare beneficiaries: site of death, place of care, and health care transitions in 2000, 2005, and 2009. JAMA. 2013;309(5):470–7.
28. Riley GF, Lubitz JD. Long-term trends in medicare payments in the last year of life. Health Serv Res. 2010;45(2):565–76.
29. Gozalo P, Plotzke M, Mor V, Miller SC, Teno JM. Changes in Medicare costs with the growth of hospice care in nursing homes. N Engl J Med. 2015;372(19):1823–31.
30. Pyenson B, Connor S, Fitch K, Kinzbrunner B. Medicare cost in matched hospice and non-hospice cohorts. J Pain Symptom Manage. 2004;28(3):200–10.
31. Campbell DE, Lynn J, Louis TA, Shugarman LR. Medicare program expenditures associated with hospice use. Ann Intern Med. 2004;140(4):269–77.
32. Obermeyer Z, Makar M, Abujaber S, Dominici F, Block S, Cutler DM. Association between the Medicare hospice benefit and health care utilization and costs for patients with poor-prognosis cancer. JAMA. 2014;312(18):1888–96.
33. Braveman P, Egerter S. Overcoming obstacles to health in 2013 and beyond. Robert Wood Johnson Foundation; 2013. http://www.rwjf.org/content/dam/farm/reports/reports/2013/rwjf406474. Cited 17 July 2015.
34. Berkowitz SA, Anderson GF. Medicare beneficiaries most likely to be readmitted. J Hosp Med. 2013;8(11):639–41.
35. Mautner DB, Pang H, Brenner JC, Shea JA, Gross KS, Frasso R, et al. Generating hypotheses about care needs of high utilizers: lessons from patient interviews. Popul Health Manag. 2013;16(S1):26–33.
36. Arbaje AI, Wolff JL, Yu Q, Powe NR, Anderson GF, Boult C. Postdischarge environmental and socioeconomic factors and the likelihood of early hospital readmission among community-dwelling Medicare beneficiaries. Gerontologist. 2008;48(4):495–504.
37. Iloabuchi TC, Mi D, Tu W, Counsell SR. Risk factors for early hospital readmission in low-income elderly adults. J Am Geriatr Soc. 2014;62(3):489–94.
38. Enguidanos S, Coulourides Kogan AM, Schreibeis-Baum H, Lendon J, Lorenz K. "Because I was sick": seriously ill veterans' perspectives on reason for 30-day readmissions. J Am Geriatr Soc. 2015;63(3):537–42.
39. Long T, Genao I, Horwitz LI. Reasons for readmission in an underserved high-risk population: a qualitative analysis of a series of inpatient interviews. BMJ Open. 2013;3(9):e003212.
40. Kansagara D, Englander H, Salanitro A, et al. Risk prediction models for hospital readmission: a systematic review. JAMA. 2011;306(15):1688–98.
41. Pacala JT, Boult C, Boult L. Predictive validity of a questionnaire that identifies older persons at risk for hospital admission. J Am Geriatr Soc. 1995;43(4):374–7.
42. Wallace E, Hinchey T, Dimitrov BD, Bennett K, Fahey T, Smith SM. A systematic review of the probability of repeated admission score in community-dwelling adults. J Am Geriatr Soc. 2013;61(3):357–64.
43. van Walraven C, Dhalla IA, Bell C, Etchells E, Stiell IG, Zarnke K, et al. Derivation and validation of an index to predict early death or unplanned readmission after discharge from hospital to the community. CMAJ. 2010;182(6):551–7.
44. Spiva L, Hand M, VanBrackle L, McVay F. Validation of a predictive model to identify patients at high risk for hospital readmission. J Healthc Qual. 2014:n/a-n/a.
45. Kind AJ, Jencks S, Brock J, Yu M, Bartels C, Ehlenbach W, et al. Neighborhood socioeconomic disadvantage and 30-day rehospitalization: a retrospective cohort study. Ann Intern Med. 2014;161(11):765–74.

46. Bowman EH, Flood KL. Care transitions intervention and other non-nursing home transitions models. In: Geriatrics Models of Care: Bringing 'Best Practice' to an Aging America, Malone ML, Capezuti EA, Palmer RM, editors. Springer International Publishing Switzerland 2015.

47. Coleman EA, Parry C, Chalmers S, Min SJ. The care transitions intervention: results of a randomized controlled trial. Arch Intern Med. 2006;166(17):1822–8.

48. Kind AJ, Jensen L, Barczi S, Bridges A, Kordahl R, Smith MA, et al. Low-cost transitional care with nurse managers making mostly phone contact with patients cut rehospitalization at a VA hospital. Health Aff (Millwood). 2012;31(12):2659–68.

49. Leppin AL, Gionfriddo MR, Kessler M, Brito JP, Mair FS, Gallacher K, et al. Preventing 30-day hospital readmissions: a systematic review and meta-analysis of randomized trials. JAMA Intern Med. 2014;174(7):1095–107.

50. Hansen LO, Young RS, Hinami K, Leung A, Williams MV. Interventions to reduce 30-day rehospitalization: a systematic review. Ann Intern Med. 2011;155(8):520–8.

51. STate Action on Avoidable Rehospitalization (STAAR). An initiative of the commonwealth fund and the Institute for Healthcare Improvement. Institute for Healthcare Improvement. 2015. www.ihi.org/staar. Cited 24 July 2015.

52. Fisher ES, McClellan MB, Bertko J, Lieberman SM, Lee JJ, Lewis JL, et al. Fostering accountable health care: moving forward in medicare. Health Aff (Millwood). 2009;28(2):w219–31.

53. Qiu WQ, Dean M, Liu T, George L, Gann M, Cohen J, et al. Physical and mental health of homebound older adults: an overlooked population. J Am Geriatr Soc. 2010;58(12):2423–8.

54. Independence at Home Demonstration Fact Sheet. Baltimore: Centers for Medicare & Medicaid Services. 2015. http://innovation.cms.gov/Files/fact-sheet/IAH-Fact-Sheet.pdf. Cited 17 July 2015.

55. Affordable Care Act payment model saves more than $25 million in first performance year (press release). Baltimore: Centers for Medicare and Medicaid Services; 2015.

56. Belluck P. Medicare plans to pay doctors for counseling on end of life. The New York Times. 2015.

57. Department of Health and Human Services Centers for Medicare & Medicaid Services. Transitional care management services: medicare learning network. 2013. https://www.acponline.org/running_practice/payment_coding/coding/tcm_factsheet.pdf. Cited 24 July 2015.

58. Goodell S, Bodenheimer TS, Berry-Millett R. Care management of patients with complex health care needs. Princeton: Robert Wood Johnson Foundation; 2009.

59. Boult C, Green AF, Boult LB, Pacala JT, Snyder C, Leff B. Successful models of comprehensive care for older adults with chronic conditions: evidence for the Institute of Medicine's "retooling for an aging America" report. J Am Geriatr Soc. 2009;57(12):2328–37.

60. Aronson L, Bautista CA, Covinsky K. Medicare and care coordination: expanding the clinician's toolbox. JAMA. 2015;313(8):797–8.

61. Medicare program; revisions to payment policies under the physician fee schedule, Clinical Laboratory Fee Schedule, access to identifiable data for the Center of Medicare and Medicaid Innovation Models & other revisions to Part B for CY 2015; Final rule. 2014. https://www.federalregister.gov/articles/2014/11/13/2014-26183/medicare-program-revisions-to-payment-policies-under-the-physician-feeschedule-clinical-laboratory. Cited 17 July 2015.

62. Medicare program; revisions to payment policies under the physician fee schedule, Clinical Laboratory Fee Schedule, access to identifiable data for the Center for Medicare and Medicaid Innovation Models & other revisions to Part B for CY 2015. https://www.federalregister.gov/articles/2014/11/13/2014-26183/medicare-program-revisions-to-payment-policies-under-the-physician-fee-schedule-clinical-laboratory. Cited 30 June 2015.

63. Edwards ST, Landon BE. Medicare's chronic care management payment — payment reform for primary care. N Engl J Med. 2014;371(22):2049–51.

64. Kindig D, Stoddart G. What is population health? Am J Public Health. 2003;93(3):380–3.

65. U.S. Department of Health and Human Services. Multiple chronic conditions- a strategic framework: optimum health and quality of life for individuals with multiple chronic conditions. Washington, DC: U.S. Department of Health and Human Services; 2010.

66. Gross K, Brenner JC, Truchil A, Post EM, Riley AH. Building a citywide, all-payer, hospital claims database to improve health care delivery in a low-income, urban community. Popul Health Manag. 2013;16(S1):20–5.
67. Brenner JC. Healthcare hotspotting 101: starting & running hotspotting interventions. Camden: The Camden Coalition; 2015.
68. Cross Site Learning: Camden Coalition of Healthcare Providers. 2015. http://www.camden-health.org/cross-site-learning/. Cited 24 July 2015.
69. Camden Coalition of Healthcare Providers. Student hotspotter mini-grant project: training the next generation of health care providers. 2015. http://www.camdenhealth.org/student-hotspotter-mini-grant-project/. Cited 24 July 2015.
70. Association of American Medical Colleges. Seeking the next generation of hot spotters!. https://www.aamc.org/download/358744/data/hotspottingguide.pdf. Cited 24 July 2015.
71. Coleman K, Austin BT, Brach C, Wagner EH. Evidence on the Chronic Care Model in the new millennium. Health Aff (Millwood). 2009;28(1):75–85.
72. Improving Chronic Illness Care. Our mission: helping the chronically ill through quality improvement and research. 2015. http://www.improvingchroniccare.org. Cited 24 July 2015
73. Friedberg MW, Schneider EC, Rosenthal MB, Volpp KG, Werner RM. Association between participation in a multipayer medical home intervention and changes in quality, utilization, and costs of care. JAMA. 2014;311(8):815–25.
74. Schwenk TL. The patient-centered medical home: one size does not fit all. JAMA. 2014;311(8):802–3.
75. Boult C, Wieland G. Comprehensive primary care for older patients with multiple chronic conditions: "nobody rushes you through". JAMA. 2010;304(17):1936–43.
76. Wieland D, Boland R, Baskins J, Kinosian B. Five-year survival in a Program of All-inclusive Care for Elderly compared with alternative institutional and home- and community-based care. J Gerontol A Biol Sci Med Sci. 2010;65(7):721–6.
77. Counsell SR, Callahan CM, Clark DO, et al. Geriatric care management for low-income seniors: a randomized controlled trial. JAMA. 2007;298(22):2623–33.
78. Counsell SR, Callahan CM, Tu W, Stump TE, Arling GW. Cost analysis of the Geriatric Resources for Assessment and Care of Elders care management intervention. J Am Geriatr Soc. 2009;57(8):1420–6.
79. Counsell SR, editor. Implementation of GRACE Team Care: a geriatrics solution for complex care management American Geriatrics Society annual scientific meeting 2015; National Harbor, MD.
80. Administration for Community Living. Administration on Aging (AoA) disease prevention and health promotion services (OAA Title IIID) (website). http://www.aoa.acl.gov/AoA_Programs/HPW/Title_IIID/index.aspx. Cited 20 July 2015.
81. National Council on Aging (NCOA). Highest tier evidence-based health promotion/disease prevention programs. https://www.ncoa.org/resources/highest-tier-evidence-based-health--promotiondisease-prevention-programs. Cited 20 July 2015.
82. Lorig KR, Sobel DS, Stewart AL, Brown Jr BW, Bandura A, Ritter P, et al. Evidence suggesting that a Chronic Disease Self-Management Program can improve health status while reducing hospitalization: a randomized trial. Med Care. 1999;37(1):5–14.
83. Ory MG, Ahn S, Jiang L, Smith ML, Ritter PL, Whitelaw N, et al. Successes of a national study of the Chronic Disease Self-Management Program: meeting the triple aim of health care reform. Med Care. 2013;51(11):992–8.
84. Stanford School of Medicine. Organizations licensed to offer the Chronic Disease Self-Management Program (CDSMP). 2015. http://patienteducation.stanford.edu/organ/cdsites.html. Cited 23 July 2015.

Challenges to Diagnosis and Management of Infections in Older Adults

3

Theresa Rowe and Geetha Iyer

Despite improvements in antibiotic therapy and vaccination rates over the past several decades, infectious diseases continue to be a major cause of morbidity and mortality among adults aged 65 and older. Approximately 30–40 % of deaths in this age group can be attributed to infectious diseases [1], and influenza, pneumonia, and septicemia are among the top 10 causes of death for older persons in the United States [2]. Hospitalization rates for infectious disease diagnoses continue to increase in the older adult population, with lower respiratory tract infections (LRTI), septicemia, urinary tract infection (UTI), and *Clostridium difficile* infection (CDI), all listed among the most common indications for hospitalization [3, 4]. Emergence of multidrug-resistant organisms (MDROs), which are more common in older adults because of increased exposure to antibiotics and repeated exposures to healthcare settings, may further lead to increasing rates of morbidity and mortality [5, 6].

Risk Factors

Several risk factors have been identified that predispose older adults to infection. Physiologic changes associated with aging, including alterations in both innate and adaptive immunity, make older adults more susceptible to developing infections

T. Rowe (✉)
Division of General Internal Medicine and Geriatrics, Northwestern University Feinberg School of Medicine, 750 N. Lake Shore Drive, 10th Floor, Chicago, IL 60611, USA
e-mail: theresa.rowe@northwestern.edu

G. Iyer
Department of Epidemiology, Johns Hopkins Bloomberg School of Public Health, 615, N Wolfe Street, Baltimore, MD 21205, USA
e-mail: giyer1@jhu.edu

© Springer International Publishing Switzerland 2016
L.A. Lindquist (ed.), *New Directions in Geriatric Medicine*,
DOI 10.1007/978-3-319-28137-7_3

[7]. These changes also lead to a reduced response to vaccination and protection against common infections such as influenza and pneumonia [8]. Multiple medical comorbidities such as diabetes mellitus and COPD, more common in older adults, increase the risk of developing an infection and often lead to a prolonged and more severe infectious course [9]. Nutritional deficiencies, particularly protein and calorie malnutrition, are associated with poor wound healing and increased risk of infection [10]. The prevalence of malnutrition is estimated to be 5–10 % of community-dwelling adults and 14 to ≥50 % of older adults residing in either a long-term care facility (LTCF) or an acute care hospital [11]. Other age-associated changes such a loss of skin integrity predispose older adults to skin and soft tissue infections [12], and poor dentition and impaired swallowing function have been shown to increase the risk of developing pneumonia [13]. Chronic urinary catheters and prosthetic devices such as joint replacements, which are most common in older adults, increase the risk of infection due to the opportunity for biofilm formation [14]. Environmental factors (i.e., residing in a LTCF or nursing home) provide an opportunity for easy transmission of highly contagious diseases such as influenza and *C. difficile*. Furthermore, repeated exposure to healthcare settings increases the risk of acquiring an infection from resistant organisms such as methicillin-resistant *Staphylococcus aureus* (MRSA), vancomycin-resistant enterococci (VRE), and extended-spectrum beta-lactamase gram-negative infections (ESBLs), which are associated with higher mortality rates [5].

Diagnostic Challenges

Prompt and accurate diagnosis of infections in older adults is challenging. Older adults, especially those with cognitive impairment, commonly present with non-specific signs and symptoms (e.g., changes in appetite, decreased functional status or mental status, agitation or delirium, and lethargy), when infected [15]. Furthermore, cardinal signs of infection (e.g., fever, leukocytosis) are less frequently observed compared to younger adults. Fever can be diminished or absent in older persons with infection, even in the setting of bacteremia [16, 17]. In LTCFs, the Infectious Disease Society of America (IDSA) defines "fever" in older adults to include a single temperature reading of ≥100 °F (37.8 °C), *or* an increase in temperature of at least 2 °F (1.1 °C) over baseline temperature, *or* a rectal temperature of ≥99.5 ° F (37.5 °C) on repeated measurements [18]. This recommendation is also frequently used for older adults living in the community [1]. Leukocytosis, another common indication for infection, can be absent, and older adults may present with a normal or lower than normal white blood cell count when infected. Lack of fever and leukocytosis in older adults with infection has been associated with increased mortality [19].

Treatment Challenges

Antibiotic prescribing in older adults presents itself with unique challenges compared to younger adults. Age-associated changes in drug absorption, distribution, metabolism, and elimination result in higher drug plasma levels and lead to an increased risk of drug toxicities and adverse drug effects [20]. Renal function is often overestimated in older adults due to declining lean muscle mass; thus, appropriate antibiotic dosing can be difficult even in older adults with a reported normal renal function [21]. Adverse reactions to antibiotics are common and one of the leading causes of emergency department (ED) visits and hospitalizations in adults aged 65 and older each year [22]. Adverse antibiotic interactions with medications such as warfarin and digoxin are also common and lead to severe adverse events including death (Table 3.1) [23].

Table 3.1 Common antibiotic side effects and significant drug interactions

Antibiotic	Side effects	Major drug interactions
Amoxicillin-clavulanate	Rash, hypersensitivity reactions, GI intolerance, and diarrhea	Allopurinol, may increase the risk of rash
Fluoroquinolones (e.g., levofloxacin, ciprofloxacin, moxifloxacin)	Tendinopathy or tendon rupture, GI intolerance, *C. difficile* colitis, photosensitivity, and QTc prolongation	Steroids, increased risk of tendinitis; warfarin, increased effect of warfarin; sucralfate or antacids, decreases absorption and efficacy; glyburide, increase risk of hyper- and hypoglycemia
Tetracyclines (e.g., doxycycline)	GI intolerance and photosensitivity	Digoxin, increased digoxin concentration; warfarin, increased effect of warfarin
Clindamycin	GI intolerance, especially diarrhea, morbilliform rash, and *C. difficile* colitis	Warfarin, increased effect of warfarin; loperamide, may increase the risk of *C. difficile* colitis
Trimethoprim-sulfamethoxazole	GI intolerance, rash and pruritus, pseudo-elevation in serum creatinine (~18 %), hyperkalemia, bone marrow suppression, photosensitivity, and hepatitis	Warfarin, increased effect of warfarin; sulfonylurea, may increase hypoglycemia
Metronidazole	GI intolerance, peripheral neuropathy (with prolonged use), and headache	Warfarin, increased effect of warfarin; alcohol, disulfiram-like reaction (acute psychosis, nausea, vomiting); lithium, increases lithium levels
Nitrofurantoin	GI intolerance, lupus-like reaction, rash, and peripheral neuropathy	Metronidazole, increases risk of peripheral neuropathy

Diagnosis and Management of Common Infections in Older Adults

Bacterial Pneumonia

Pneumonia is one of the most serious infections in adults aged ≥65 years and is the fifth leading cause of death in this age group [2]. Older residents of LTCFs have an even higher risk of developing pneumonia with an incident rate of 1.8–13.5 infections per 100 resident-care days [24]. Pneumonia is generally divided into several categories based on location of symptom onset [25]:

- Community-acquired pneumonia (CAP) is defined as pneumonia occurring in community-dwelling adults.
- Hospital-acquired pneumonia (HAP) is defined as pneumonia that occurs ≥48 h after an acute hospital admission without evidence of infection upon admission to the hospital.
- Healthcare-associated pneumonia (HCAP) is defined as pneumonia that occurs in a nonhospitalized adult with extensive healthcare contact (e.g., receiving intravenous therapy including chemotherapy, receiving wound care, residence in LTCF, hospitalization for ≥2 days within 90 days, or attendance at hospital or hemodialysis clinic with 30 days of symptom onset).
- Nursing home-acquired pneumonia falls under the definition of HCAP, limiting the population to nursing home or LTCF residents.

Epidemiology

Organisms causative of pneumonia in older adults are different than younger adults, although there is significant variability in the literature. The most common cause of bacterial pneumonia in older adults is *Streptococcus pneumoniae* (*S. pneumoniae*), followed by *Haemophilus influenzae* (*H. influenzae*), *Staphylococcus aureus* (*S. aureus*), *Moraxella catarrhalis*, and other gram-negative rods including *Pseudomonas aeruginosa* [26]. *Chlamydia pneumonia*, *Mycoplasma pneumonia*, and *Legionella* species have also been implicated, although are less frequently documented in older adults compared to younger adults [27]. Older adults with impaired swallowing function are at risk for developing aspiration pneumonia, which is often a polymicrobial infection. In community-acquired cases, infection usually involves *Streptococcus* species and anaerobes, while in hospital-acquired cases, *S. aureus* and gram-negative infections predominate [28]. Identifying the exact etiology of pneumonia is challenging in older adults because of difficulty in obtaining an adequate sputum culture. Urinary antigen testing for *S. pneumoniae*, which has sensitivity rates of approximately 80 % for detecting *S. pneumoniae*, has increased the number of confirmed cases of streptococcal pneumonia [29].

The most significant risk factor for pneumonia is the presence of comorbidity, particularly cancer, collagen vascular disease, liver disease, and COPD [30]. Other factors include older age, male sex, swallowing dysfunction, witnessed aspiration, poor baseline functional status, residence in a LTCF, and inability to take oral medications [13, 26, 30]. In a cohort of older adults hospitalized with CAP, hospital mortality doubled with age from 7.8 % in those aged 65–69 years to 15.4 % in those aged ≥90 years [26]. Medications such as sedatives, H2 receptor blockers, proton pump inhibitors, antipsychotics, and anticholinergics have also been shown to increase the risk of developing pneumonia [31].

Diagnosis and Treatment

Diagnosis and treatment of pneumonia in older adults generally depends on place of residence (e.g., LTCF vs. community setting), risk factors for resistant organisms, and the presence of comorbidities. According to IDSA guidelines, CAP in adults aged 60 and older should be treated with a beta lactam/beta lactamase (e.g., amoxicillin-clavulanate or ceftriaxone) plus either doxycycline or a macrolide (e.g., azithromycin). Alternative therapy includes respiratory fluoroquinolones (e.g., moxifloxacin, levofloxacin) [32]. Healthcare providers, however, should be cautious with use of fluoroquinolones in frail older adults because of the risk of Achilles tendon rupture and cardiac arrhythmias in this age group. In HAP, HCAP, or where resistant organisms are suspected, coverage should additionally include treatment for MRSA with either linezolid or vancomycin. Daptomycin should not be used to cover MRSA pneumonia because it is inactivated by lung surfactant, and treatment failure has been reported. In cases of suspected aspiration pneumonia, treatment with clindamycin is preferred given the high likelihood of infection with anaerobes [32].

The most evidence-based intervention for pneumonia prevention is vaccination for both pneumococcus and influenza. Other potential prevention measures include maintaining adequate oral hygiene, limiting use of sedating medications, and providing interventions that improve mobility [33].

Pneumococcal Vaccination

Pneumococcal vaccination with the 23-valent pneumococcal polysaccharide vaccine (PPSV23) has been shown to be effective for preventing invasive pneumococcal disease, particularly bacteremia, in adults aged 65 years and older [34]. However, the efficacy of PPSV23 in preventing pneumococcal pneumonia in this population is not as well established. In 2014, the Centers for Disease Control and Prevention (CDC) began recommending the 13-valent pneumococcal conjugate vaccine (PCV13), previously only given to younger children, for use in adults aged ≥65 years, after a randomized placebo-controlled trial demonstrated efficacy against vaccine-type CAP (45 %) and vaccine-type invasive disease (75 %), in this population [35]. The Advisory Committee on Immunization Practices (ACIP) now recommends PCV13 followed by PPSV23 (6–12 months apart) in adults aged ≥65 years who have never received a pneumococcal vaccination. If PPSV23 has already been given, PCV13 should be given ≥1 year after PPSV23. The two vaccinations should never be given together because of decreased effectiveness of the vaccines. Immunization of PCV13 to children has also been shown to reduce the incidence of pneumococcal pneumonia in older adults, possibly by herd immunity [36].

Influenza

Influenza is a common cause of acute respiratory disease among older adults and is highly contagious. Influenza is responsible 36,000 deaths and 226,000 hospitalizations per year in the United States [37, 38]. Infection rates can vary year to year, depending on the effectiveness of the influenza vaccine and the virulence of circulating flu strain. Although symptoms of influenza are similar to those of bacterial pneumonia in older adults, abrupt onset of high fevers, chills, myalgias, and sore throat during the influenza season (September–April) should heighten suspicion of influenza infection. Prompt diagnosis and treatment of influenza is vital because of rapid spread of disease and high mortality rates in this population. Neuraminidase inhibitors (e.g., oseltamivir) are effective against influenza A and B if started within 24–48 h of symptom onset and can also be used to prevent influenza during outbreaks, especially in LTCFs or acute care hospitals. M2 inhibitors (amantadine) are no longer recommended for treatment of influenza because of high resistance rates and severe CNS side effects including increased confusion and seizures. Treatment with antivirals should not be delayed while awaiting diagnostic testing for influenza. A serious complication of influenza infection is subsequent or concurrent bacterial pneumonia, most common in older adults with underlying comorbidities such as diabetes or COPD. The most common pathogens associated with secondary bacterial pneumonia are *S. aureus* (including MRSA) and group A *Streptococcus*.

Influenza Vaccination

Influenza vaccination is one of the most important prevention strategies available for reducing morbidity and mortality from influenza infection in older adults. Recently, the FDA approved a high-dose influenza vaccine, which contains four times the amount of hemagglutinin (antigen) as the standard dose vaccine, for the use in adults aged 65 years and older. The FDA approval was based on previous studies that showed improved immune responses to the higher dose vaccine in adults ≥65 years [39]. A recent randomized controlled study confirmed that the high-dose vaccination improved protection against laboratory confirmed influenza illness in adults aged 65 and older compared to the standard dose vaccine with a relative efficacy of 24.2 % (CI 9.7–36.5) [37]. The ACIP now recommends the high-dose inactivated influenza vaccines for adults aged 65 years and older.

Urinary Tract Infection and Asymptomatic Bacteriuria

Urinary tract infection (UTI) is the most commonly diagnosed bacterial infection in adults aged 65 years and older in both the community and healthcare settings [40]. The definition of symptomatic UTI includes the presence of localized genitourinary signs or symptoms plus pyuria defined as ≥10 white blood cells per high power field (wbc/hpf) and bacteriuria defined as $\geq 10^5$ colony-forming units per milliliter (CFU/mL). Asymptomatic bacteriuria (ASB) is generally defined as bacteriuria in the absence of genitourinary signs and symptoms of infection. It is important to distinguish symptomatic UTI from ASB, as the former requires treatment with antimicrobial therapy.

Asymptomatic Bacteriuria

ASB is common and present in up to 30 % of community-dwelling older adults and up to 50 % of adults living in LTCFs [41]. In men, the formal definition of ASB is defined as one voided urine specimen with $\geq 10^5$ colony-forming units/milliliter (CFU/mL) of 1 uropathogen without the presence of genitourinary signs or symptoms of infection. In women, ASB is defined as two consecutive urine specimens positive for the same uropathogen in quantities $\geq 10^5$ CFU/mL without the presence of genitourinary signs or symptoms of infection. A single catheterized urine specimen with 1 uropathogen in quantities $\geq 10^5$ CFU/mL without the presence of genitourinary signs or symptoms of infection defines ASB in both men and women. Multiple studies have shown no benefit to treating ASB; thus, routine screening and use of antibiotics are not recommended for asymptomatic older adults. Screening and treatment for ASB may be indicated in men before transurethral resection of the prostate and for men and women undergoing a urologic procedure for which there may be mucosal bleeding [42]. Inappropriate use of antibiotics for treatment of ASB continues to be a significant healthcare problem and leads to the development of resistant organism.

Symptomatic Urinary Tract Infection

Symptomatic UTI, in contrast to ASB, does require treatment with antimicrobials. The most common cause of symptomatic UTI in older adults is *Escherichia coli* (*E. coli*) followed by other Enterobacteriaceae, such as *Proteus mirabilis*, *Klebsiella* species, *Providencia*, and *Pseudomonas* species [43]. Risk factors for symptomatic UTI include having a prior history of UTI [44], presence of comorbidities such as cerebrovascular disease and dementia [45], prostatic hypertrophy in men, vaginal atrophy in women, and the presence of a urinary catheter [46]. Diagnosis and treatment of symptomatic UTI in cognitively intact community-dwelling older adults is similar to younger adults and includes the presence signs or symptoms of a genitourinary tract infection (e.g., new or worsening urgency, frequency, suprapubic pain, gross hematuria), plus pyuria and bacteriuria [47]. In older adults who have cognitive impairment and those living in LTCFs, the diagnosis is more challenging because of the variability in presenting signs and symptoms of infection and the inability to communicate the presence of specific genitourinary symptoms [15]. In 2012 the CDC along with the Society for Healthcare Epidemiology of America (SHEA) updated consensus criteria for diagnosis of symptomatic UTI in residents of LTCFs in attempt to prevent unnecessary use of antimicrobials [48]. According to the updated guidelines, diagnosis of symptomatic UTI in residents without an indwelling urinary catheter should include:

1. Swelling or tenderness of the testes, epididymis, or prostate
2. Fever or leukocytosis and at least one of the following:

- Acute costovertebral angle pain or tenderness
- Suprapubic pain
- Gross hematuria
- New or marked increase in incontinence
- New or marked increase in urgency or frequency
3. In the absence of fever and leukocytosis at least two of the following:
   - Suprapubic pain
   - Gross hematuria
   - New or marked increase in incontinence
   - New or marked increase in urgency
   - New or marked increase in frequency

plus a positive urine culture for a uropathogen $\geq 10^5$ CFU/mL

Diagnosis of symptomatic UTI in residents without an indwelling urinary catheter should include:

1. At least one of the following criteria:
   (a) Fever, rigors, or new-onset hypotension
   (b) Acute change in mental status or acute functional decline and leukocytosis
   (c) New-onset suprapubic pain or costovertebral angle pain or tenderness
   (d) Purulent discharge from around the catheter or acute pain, swelling or tenderness of the testes, epididymis, or prostate

plus a positive urine culture for a uropathogen $\geq 10^5$ CFU/mL

Although these guidelines have been adapted by several professional societies and LTCF administrations, the use by clinicians and other healthcare providers remains low [49]. This often leads to overuse of antibiotics for suspected UTI in this population [50]. Some experts recommend use of urinary dipstick testing to evaluate for the presence of leukocyte esterase and nitrites, as the first step in older adults suspected of having a symptomatic UTI. A urinary dipstick negative for both leukocyte esterase and nitrate has an excellent negative predictive value (88–100 %) for bacteriuria. Thus, a negative test can help rule out symptomatic UTI [51]. The presence of leukocyte esterase and/or nitrates, however, does not confirm the diagnosis of UTI and further testing with urinalysis and urine culture is needed.

Treatment for symptomatic UTI in older adults is similar to younger adults and based on the International Clinical Practice Guidelines, issued in 2010 by IDSA and the European Society of Clinical Microbiology and Infectious Diseases [52]. First-line recommendations include nitrofurantoin monohydrate/macrocrystals 100 mg twice daily for 5 days or trimethoprim-sulfamethoxazole 160/800 mg twice daily for 3 days, if local resistance rates do not exceed 20 %. Nitrofurantoin, however, is contraindicated in adults with chronic kidney disease who have a creatinine clearance ≤ 60 mL/min, although few studies have demonstrated efficacy and safety in adults with a creatinine clearance of ≥ 40 mL/min [53]. Nitrofurantoin is also not recommended if upper urinary tract disease (e.g., pyelonephritis) or if bacteremia is suspected. Furthermore, non-*E. coli* pathogens (e.g., *Klebsiella* spp., *Proteus* spp.)

have higher resistant rates to nitrofurantoin, making it a less-appealing choice for older adults who have higher rates of UTI caused by other Enterobacteriaceae. The use of fluoroquinolones, although commonly prescribed for symptomatic UTI in this population, is not recommended because of high resistance rates across multiple geographic areas [54]. However, they can be used if laboratory testing confirms sensitivity.

Prevention of recurrent UTI in older adults includes both antimicrobial prophylaxis and non-antimicrobial therapies (e.g., cranberry formulations, vaginal estrogens, lactobacilli). In general, prophylaxis with antibiotics is not routinely recommended because of the limited data to support their use in prevention of UTI and the high risk of developing antibiotic resistance. Intravaginal estrogen replacement has been shown in few small studies to reduce the incidence of recurrent UTI, although oral estrogens have not been shown to be beneficial [55]. Cranberry-containing products may reduce the incidence of bacteriuria in nursing home residents [56], although the evidence for use in community-dwelling older adults is not well established [57] .

Skin and Soft Tissue Infections

Invasion of the skin and soft tissues by microorganisms result in infections, often presenting with variable severity. Skin and soft tissue infections (SSTI) are common in older adults and have been consistently increasing over the past decade [58, 59]. SSTIs range from mild non-purulent infections (e.g., cellulitis) to life-threatening conditions such as necrotizing fasciitis that require emergent surgical intervention.

Epidemiology

Cellulitis is an acute inflammatory condition of the skin and underlying soft tissue (i.e., involving the dermis and subcutaneous tissue) and is the most common cause of SSTI in older adults. Cellulitis is generally categorized as purulent and non-purulent based on the etiologic organism. Purulent cellulitis is associated with purulent drainage or exudate in the absence of a drainable abscess, whereas non-purulent cellulitis is defined as a skin and soft tissue infection without purulent drainage. Non-purulent cellulitis is most often caused by beta-hemolytic streptococci and purulent cellulitis by *S. aureus* [60]. The emergence of MRSA has led to increasing rates of purulent cellulitis in adults [58]. Gram-negative organisms such as *E. coli*, *Pseudomonas* spp., and *Enterococcus* spp. are rarer causes of SSTI, although they can be diagnosed in older adults with immunocompromising conditions [61]. The older adult population is at greater risk for developing cellulitis and other SSTIs compared to the general population for a variety of reasons. Chronic skin conditions such as lymphedema, venous stasis, eczema, and psoriasis increase the risk of developing a SSTI. Uncontrolled diabetes (HgA1C >8 %), congestive heart failure, history of chemotherapy, the use of immunosuppressants or corticosteroid therapy, and malnutrition, more common in older adults, are all risk factors for developing a SSTI [62].

Diagnosis and Treatment

The diagnosis of cellulitis is clinical and typically presents with pain, localized erythema, and swelling of the involved skin and subcutaneous tissues [64]. These features can be associated with systemic symptoms such as fever (temperature >38 °C), tachycardia (heart rate >90 beats per minute), tachypnea (respiratory rate >24 breaths per minute), or abnormal white blood cell count (>12,000 or <400 white blood cells/μL). It is important to differentiate cellulitis from other inflammatory conditions which often mimic cellulitis. Conditions such as bursitis, gout, hypersensitivity drug reactions, contact dermatitis, herpes zoster, and venous stasis can present with localized erythema and swelling, but do not require antimicrobial therapy. Prompt diagnosis of more severe SSTI such as necrotizing fasciitis, and acute septic arthritis, is vital as these conditions often require emergent surgical treatment. The presence of severe pain, clinical instability (toxic appearing, hypotension, and tachycardia), the presence of hemorrhagic bullae, and evidence of skin necrosis or crepitus on clinical examination should prompt consideration of a more severe infection.

According to the 2014 IDSA guidelines, adults diagnosed with cellulitis who do not have systemic signs of infection may be treatment with a beta-lactam antibiotic (e.g., oral amoxicillin, cephalexin, or clindamycin if penicillin allergic). Intravenous treatment can also be given if systemic signs of infection are present. For patients with purulent cellulitis in which MRSA is suspected, oral trimethoprim-sulfamethoxazole or linezolid, or intravenous vancomycin, or daptomycin is preferred. For hospitalized older adults with a severe infection, vancomycin plus either piperacillin-tazobactam or imipenem-meropenem is a reasonable empiric choice. In addition to antibiotic therapy, older adults with cellulitis should be encouraged to elevate the affected area, and treatment of predisposing factors (e.g., edema or underlying cutaneous disorders) should be initiated [60].

Herpes Zoster

Herpes zoster infection (shingles) is a reactivation of the varicella-zoster virus that remains latent in the dorsal root ganglia after an initial infection (i.e., chicken pox). Older adults have the highest risk of infection, about 20 % in those aged 60 years and older. Shingles typically presents as a unilateral vesicular eruption that follows a dermatomal distribution and can be accompanied by pain, paresthesias, and/or pruritus. Diagnosis can usually be made by clinical exam alone, although vesicles can be swabbed and sent for PCR analysis to confirm diagnosis. Treatment with antivirals (e.g., valacyclovir, famciclovir) is most effective if used within 72 h of rash onset [63]. Treatment has been shown to decrease the severity of acute pain, but not to lessen the risk of developing post-herpetic neuralgia (neuropathic pain persisting after resolution of rash) [64]. Ophthalmology should always be consulted if there is concern for eye involvement, as herpes zoster ophthalmicus can lead to acute retinal necrosis and blindness.

Herpes Zoster Vaccination

Herpes zoster vaccination, commonly known as Zostavax, is a live attenuated virus vaccine recommended by ACIP for prevention of herpes zoster in adults aged ≥60 years old, including those with a prior history of herpes zoster infection. A large study evaluating the efficacy of herpes zoster vaccination in adults aged ≥60 years old reported a reduced incidence of herpes zoster by 51.3 % (95 % CI, 47.5–79.2) in adults who received the vaccination compared to placebo [65]. More recently, a follow-up study confirmed ongoing vaccine efficacy of 39.6 % (95 % CI, 18.2–55.2) for up to 5 years postvaccination [66]. The vaccine has also been shown to decrease the incidence of post-herpetic neuralgia and duration of pain and discomfort in those who develop an active infection. Because the vaccination is a live virus vaccine, older adults with primary or acquired immunodeficiencies should not receive the vaccine.

Clostridium difficile Infection

Clostridium difficile infection (CDI) is the most common healthcare-acquired infection, predominately affecting older adults. A recent study describes that over half of CDI in the United States are in adults aged 65 years and older with an incidence estimated to be 627.7 per 100,000 persons in this age group. Furthermore, CDI accounts for an estimated 24,000 deaths in adults aged ≥65 years and is listed as the 18th leading cause of death in this population [67]. Age, healthcare exposure, and antibiotic use are the most significant risk factors for developing CDI. Older age (>70 years old) has also been shown to be a risk factor for more severe disease [68]. Older adults residing in LTCFs are increased risk for developing CDI for a variety of factors including increased proximity to other residents and increased exposure to antibiotics. A study in LTCFs in New York describes that over half of CDI have occurred in LTCF residents more than 4 weeks after hospital discharge, suggesting CDI in LTCFs is as common as those occurring in the hospital setting [69].

The presentation of CDI in older adults usually involves watery diarrhea and abdominal cramping; fever may be present or absent. Significant leukocytosis (>20,000 WBC/µL) can also be seen, even in older adults. The definition of CDI is based on a combination of clinical and laboratory findings including (1) diarrhea defined as ≥3 unformed stools in <24 h and (2) positive laboratory result for *C. difficile* or (3) colonoscopic or histopathologic findings consistent with pseudo-membranous colitis [70]. The most sensitive test for CDI is polymerase chain reaction for toxin B gene. However, this may also pick up "carrier" cases and, thus, should only be performed on unformed stool and not in asymptomatic older adults. Enzyme immunoassay testing (EIA) followed by toxin A and B assay is also used, although it is a less sensitive test.

The most important aspect of treatment for CDI is discontinuing offending antibiotics. If antibiotics cannot be discontinued, the potential use of a more narrow-spectrum antibiotic should be explored. Treatment for CDI does not vary with age and largely depends on the severity of disease. Per IDSA/SHEA guidelines, severe illness is defined as (1) WBC count ≥15,000/µL or (2) serum creatinine level >1.5 times baseline creatinine or (3) evidence of ileus. Severe infection should be treated with oral vancomycin 125 mg every 6 h for 10–14 days. For mild to moderate disease, IDSA recommends metronidazole 500 mg every 8 h for 10–14 days (Table 3.2) [70]. Repeated testing for *C. difficile* during the same episode of diarrhea and a "test of cure" should never be obtained. Response to treatment should be monitored clinically. Antiperistaltic medications (e.g., loperamide) should not be given during infection due to the possible increased risk of developing complications such as toxic megacolon or colonic distention, although the evidence for this is minimal

Table 3.2 Treatment for *Clostridium difficile* infection in older adults

Severity	Definition	Treatment
Asymptomatic carrier	No signs or symptoms of infection	Do not treat
Initial episode, mild to moderate	• Diarrhea (>3 unformed bowel movements <24 h) • WBC <15,000 • Creatinine <1.5 times baseline	• Metronidazole, 500 mg orally three times per day for 10–14 days
Initial episode, severe	• WBC > 15,000 • Creatinine > 1.5 times baseline • Albumin level <3 mg/dL • Temperature > 38.9 °C	• Vancomycin, 125 mg orally four times per day for 10–14 days
Initial episode, severe with evidence of ileus	• WBC > 15,000 • Creatinine > 1.5 times baseline • Albumin level <3 mg/dL • Temperature > 38.9 °C • Ileus	• Vancomycin, 500 mg orally four times per day (and per rectum if ileus is present), ± intravenous metronidazole 800 mg three times per day
Complicated	• Toxic megacolon • Hemodynamic instability	• Vancomycin, 500 mg orally four times per day, ± intravenous metronidazole 800 mg three times per day • Surgical consultation
First recurrence	• New onset of symptoms <8 weeks after the onset of the previous episode, assuming symptoms from the prior episode had resolved	• Same as initial episode, although consider vancomycin, if recurrence is more severe (even in those who received metronidazole)
Second recurrence	• >1 recurrence as defined above	• Vancomycin, 125 mg orally four times daily, tapered over several weeks *or* • Fidaxomicin 200 mg orally twice daily for 10 days • Consider fecal microbial transplantation

[71]. For recurrent or prolonged cases of CDI in older adults, a vancomycin taper may be needed (Table 3.2). A recurrent episode of CDI is defined as an episode of CDI that occurs <8 weeks after the onset of the previous episode, assuming symptoms from the prior episode had resolved. Fidaxomicin 200 mg twice daily has been shown to reduce the rate of relapse compared to vancomycin; however, the cost of this medication often limits the use in most clinical settings. Other supportive measures such as maintaining adequate hydration (oral or intravenously) and replacement of electrolytes are often necessary, particularly in frail older adults (Table 3.3).

Prevention of CDI is extremely important and involves a multidisciplinary approach both to decrease the risk of transmission and to reduce susceptibility of infection by limiting unnecessary antibiotic use. Healthcare workers (e.g., RNs, MDs, CNAs, etc.) and visitors must follow appropriate contact precautions (e.g., gloves and gown) upon entering the room of a resident with CDI. Everyone who enters/leaves the room should wash their hands with soap and warm water.

Table 3.3 Review of infections, their risk factors, and treatment

Infection	Risk factors	Points to consider while managing the patient
Bacterial pneumonia	• Male gender • Comorbidities such as COPD and cancer • Swallowing dysfunction • Inability to take oral medications • Witnessed aspiration	• Consider influenza during flu season (September to April) • Ensure pneumococcal (PCV13 and PPSV23) and influenza vaccination are given
Urinary tract infection	• Previous history of UTI • Presence of indwelling catheter • Presence of comorbidities such as dementia and diabetes mellitus • Prostatic hypertrophy in men	• Do not treat asymptomatic bacteriuria • Avoid empiric use of fluoroquinolones unless sensitivity results are known
Cellulitis	• Lymphedema or venous stasis • Preexisting skin conditions such as psoriasis and eczema • History of diabetes mellitus, congestive heart failure, and immunosuppressants	• Consider differential diagnosis of conditions that mimic cellulitis • Exclude necrotizing fasciitis as a possible diagnosis • Look for signs and symptoms suggestive of MRSA infection (e.g., purulent drainage)
Clostridium difficile infection	• Regular exposure to healthcare systems • Exposure to broad-spectrum antibiotics • Residence in a long-term care facility	• Discontinue offending antibiotics • Do not prescribe antiperistaltic drugs (e.g. loperamide) • Encourage strict contact precautions in all confirmed cases

C. difficile spores are resistant to antibacterial gels; thus, antibacterial gels and creams should not be used for hand hygiene practices in adults with CDI. Hospitalized patients and residents of LTCFs with CDI should be moved to a private room, if possible. IDSA recommends that environmental services use chlorine-containing cleaning agents to clean room surfaces and use disposable equipment (e.g., thermometers, stethoscopes), if possible. Antibiotic stewardship programs that help minimize the use and frequency of antibiotics are of utmost importance for prevention of CDI.

Key Points
1. Infections may present atypically in older adults, and cardinal signs of infection such as fever and leukocytosis are often absent.
2. Pneumococcal conjugate vaccination (PCV13) is now recommended in adults aged 65 years and older after a recent study demonstrated efficacy against vaccine-type community-acquired pneumococcal pneumonia and vaccine-type invasive pneumococcal disease.
3. Distinguishing between asymptomatic bacteriuria and symptomatic urinary tract infection is important, as asymptomatic bacteriuria does not require treatment with antibiotics.
4. Prevention of *Clostridium difficile* infection in older adults involves both reducing susceptibility to infection by reducing the number of unnecessary antibiotics and minimizing transmission of disease, especially in the hospital and long-term care setting. (Table 3.3) is a review of the most common infections, their risk factors, and treatment.

References

1. Mouton CP, Bazaldua OV, Pierce B, Espino DV. Common infections in older adults. Am Fam Physician. 2001;63(2):257–68.
2. Gorina YHD, Lentzner H, Goulding M. Trends in causes of death among older persons in the United States, Aging trends, vol. 6. Hyattsville: National Center for Health Statistics; 2006.
3. Christensen KL, Holman RC, Steiner CA, Sejvar JJ, Stoll BJ, Schonberger LB. Infectious disease hospitalizations in the United States. Clin Infect Dis. 2009;49(7):1025–35.
4. Curns AT, Holman RC, Sejvar JJ, Owings MF, Schonberger LB. Infectious disease hospitalizations among older adults in the United States from 1990 through 2002. Arch Intern Med. 2005;165(21):2514–20.
5. Pop-Vicas A, Tacconelli E, Gravenstein S, Lu B, D'Agata EM. Influx of multidrug-resistant, gram-negative bacteria in the hospital setting and the role of elderly patients with bacterial bloodstream infection. Infect Control Hosp Epidemiol. 2009;30(4):325–31.
6. Yoshikawa TT. Antimicrobial resistance and aging: beginning of the end of the antibiotic era? J Am Geriatr Soc. 2002;50(7 Suppl):S226–9.
7. Gomez CR, Boehmer ED, Kovacs EJ. The aging innate immune system. Curr Opin Immunol. 2005;17(5):457–62.
8. Goodwin K, Viboud C, Simonsen L. Antibody response to influenza vaccination in the elderly: a quantitative review. Vaccine. 2006;24(8):1159–69.

9. Bertoni AG, Saydah S, Brancati FL. Diabetes and the risk of infection-related mortality in the U.S. Diabetes Care. 2001;24(6):1044–9.
10. Katona P, Katona-Apte J. The interaction between nutrition and infection. Clin Infect Dis. 2008;46(10):1582–8.
11. Kaiser MJ, Bauer JM, Ramsch C, Uter W, Guigoz Y, Cederholm T, et al. Frequency of malnutrition in older adults: a multinational perspective using the mini nutritional assessment. J Am Geriatr Soc. 2010;58(9):1734–8.
12. Compton GA. Bacterial skin and soft tissue infections in older adults. Clin Geriatr Med. 2013;29(2):443–59.
13. Quagliarello V, Ginter S, Han L, Van Ness P, Allore H, Tinetti M. Modifiable risk factors for nursing home-acquired pneumonia. Clin Infect Dis. 2005;40(1):1–6.
14. Donlan RM. Biofilm formation: a clinically relevant microbiological process. Clin Infect Dis. 2001;33(8):1387–92.
15. D'Agata E, Loeb MB, Mitchell SL. Challenges in assessing nursing home residents with advanced dementia for suspected urinary tract infections. J Am Geriatr Soc. 2013; 61(1):62–6.
16. Norman DC. Fever in the elderly. Clin Infect Dis. 2000;31(1):148–51.
17. Gleckman R, Hibert D. Afebrile bacteremia. A phenomenon in geriatric patients. JAMA. 1982;248(12):1478–81.
18. High KP, Bradley SF, Gravenstein S, Mehr DR, Quagliarello VJ, Richards C, et al. Clinical practice guideline for the evaluation of fever and infection in older adult residents of long-term care facilities: 2008 update by the Infectious Diseases Society of America. Clin Infect Dis. 2009;48(2):149–71.
19. Ahkee S, Srinath L, Ramirez J. Community-acquired pneumonia in the elderly: association of mortality with lack of fever and leukocytosis. South Med J. 1997;90(3):296–8.
20. Faulkner CM, Cox HL, Williamson JC. Unique aspects of antimicrobial use in older adults. Clin Infect Dis. 2005;40(7):997–1004.
21. Drusano GL, Munice Jr HL, Hoopes JM, Damron DJ, Warren JW. Commonly used methods of estimating creatinine clearance are inadequate for elderly debilitated nursing home patients. J Am Geriatr Soc. 1988;36(5):437–41.
22. Budnitz DS, Shehab N, Kegler SR, Richards CL. Medication use leading to emergency department visits for adverse drug events in older adults. Ann Intern Med. 2007;147(11):755–65.
23. Shehab N, Patel PR, Srinivasan A, Budnitz DS. Emergency department visits for antibiotic-associated adverse events. Clin Infect Dis. 2008;47(6):735–43.
24. Strausbaugh LJ, Joseph CL. The burden of infection in long-term care. Infect Control Hosp Epidemiol. 2000;21(10):674–9.
25. Anand N, Kollef MH. The alphabet soup of pneumonia: CAP, HAP, HCAP, NHAP, and VAP. Semin Respir Crit Care Med. 2009;30(1):3–9.
26. Kaplan V, Angus DC, Griffin MF, Clermont G, Scott Watson R, Linde-Zwirble WT. Hospitalized community-acquired pneumonia in the elderly: age- and sex-related patterns of care and outcome in the United States. Am J Respir Crit Care Med. 2002;165(6):766–72.
27. Loeb M. Pneumonia in older persons. Clin Infect Dis. 2003;37(10):1335–9.
28. Marik PE. Aspiration pneumonitis and aspiration pneumonia. N Engl J Med. 2001; 344(9):665–71.
29. Smith MD, Derrington P, Evans R, Creek M, Morris R, Dance DA, et al. Rapid diagnosis of bacteremic pneumococcal infections in adults by using the Binax NOW *Streptococcus pneumoniae* urinary antigen test: a prospective, controlled clinical evaluation. J Clin Microbiol. 2003;41(7):2810–3.
30. Jackson ML, Neuzil KM, Thompson WW, Shay DK, Yu O, Hanson CA, et al. The burden of community-acquired pneumonia in seniors: results of a population-based study. Clin Infect Dis. 2004;39(11):1642–50.
31. Vergis EN, Brennen C, Wagener M, Muder RR. Pneumonia in long-term care: a prospective case–control study of risk factors and impact on survival. Arch Intern Med. 2001;161(19): 2378–81.

32. Mandell LA, Wunderink RG, Anzueto A, Bartlett JG, Campbell GD, Dean NC, et al. Infectious Diseases Society of America/American Thoracic Society consensus guidelines on the management of community-acquired pneumonia in adults. Clin Infect Dis. 2007;44 Suppl 2:S27–72.
33. Juthani-Mehta M, De Rekeneire N, Allore H, Chen S, O'Leary JR, Bauer DC, et al. Modifiable risk factors for pneumonia requiring hospitalization of community-dwelling older adults: the Health, Aging, and Body Composition Study. J Am Geriatr Soc. 2013;61(7):1111–8.
34. Moberley S, Holden J, Tatham DP, Andrews RM. Vaccines for preventing pneumococcal infection in adults. Cochrane Database Syst Rev. 2013;(1):CD000422.
35. Bonten MJ, Huijts SM, Bolkenbaas M, Webber C, Patterson S, Gault S, et al. Polysaccharide conjugate vaccine against pneumococcal pneumonia in adults. N Engl J Med. 2015; 372(12):1114–25.
36. Lexau CA, Lynfield R, Danila R, Pilishvili T, Facklam R, Farley MM, et al. Changing epidemiology of invasive pneumococcal disease among older adults in the era of pediatric pneumococcal conjugate vaccine. JAMA. 2005;294(16):2043–51.
37. DiazGranados CA, Dunning AJ, Kimmel M, Kirby D, Treanor J, Collins A, et al. Efficacy of high-dose versus standard-dose influenza vaccine in older adults. N Engl J Med. 2014; 371(7):635–45.
38. Fiore AE, Uyeki TM, Broder K, Finelli L, Euler GL, Singleton JA, et al. Prevention and control of influenza with vaccines: recommendations of the Advisory Committee on Immunization Practices (ACIP), 2010. MMWR Recomm Rep. 2010;59(RR-8):1–62.
39. DiazGranados CA, Dunning AJ, Jordanov E, Landolfi V, Denis M, Talbot HK. High-dose trivalent influenza vaccine compared to standard dose vaccine in elderly adults: safety, immunogenicity and relative efficacy during the 2009–2010 season. Vaccine. 2013;31(6):861–6.
40. Schappert SM, Rechtsteiner EA. Ambulatory medical care utilization estimates for 2007. Vital Health Stat 13, Data from the National Health Survey. 2011;(169):1–38.
41. Juthani-Mehta M. Asymptomatic bacteriuria and urinary tract infection in older adults. Clin Geriatr Med. 2007;23(3):585–94.
42. Nicolle LE, Bradley S, Colgan R, Rice JC, Schaeffer A, Hooton TM, et al. Infectious Diseases Society of America guidelines for the diagnosis and treatment of asymptomatic bacteriuria in adults. Clin Infect Dis. 2005;40(5):643–54.
43. Das R, Perrelli E, Towle V, Van Ness PH, Juthani-Mehta M. Antimicrobial susceptibility of bacteria isolated from urine samples obtained from nursing home residents. Infect Control Hosp Epidemiol. 2009;30(11):1116–9.
44. Jackson SL, Boyko EJ, Scholes D, Abraham L, Gupta K, Fihn SD. Predictors of urinary tract infection after menopause: a prospective study. Am J Med. 2004;117(12):903–11.
45. Caljouw MA, den Elzen WP, Cools HJ, Gussekloo J. Predictive factors of urinary tract infections among the oldest old in the general population. A population-based prospective follow-up study. BMC Med. 2011;9:57.
46. Nicolle LE. Urinary tract infections in the elderly. Clin Geriatr Med. 2009;25(3):423–36.
47. Hooton TM. Clinical practice. Uncomplicated urinary tract infection. N Engl J Med. 2012;366(11):1028–37.
48. Stone ND, Ashraf MS, Calder J, Crnich CJ, Crossley K, Drinka PJ, et al. Surveillance definitions of infections in long-term care facilities: revisiting the McGeer criteria. Infect Control Hosp Epidemiol. 2012;33(10):965–77.
49. Juthani-Mehta M, Drickamer MA, Towle V, Zhang Y, Tinetti ME, Quagliarello VJ. Nursing home practitioner survey of diagnostic criteria for urinary tract infections. J Am Geriatr Soc. 2005;53(11):1986–90.
50. Olsho LE, Bertrand RM, Edwards AS, Hadden LS, Morefield GB, Hurd D, et al. Does adherence to the Loeb minimum criteria reduce antibiotic prescribing rates in nursing homes? J Am Med Dir Assoc. 2013;14(4):309.e1–7.
51. Juthani-Mehta M, Tinetti M, Perrelli E, Towle V, Quagliarello V. Role of dipstick testing in the evaluation of urinary tract infection in nursing home residents. Infect Control Hosp Epidemiol. 2007;28(7):889–91.

52. Gupta K, Hooton TM, Naber KG, Wullt B, Colgan R, Miller LG, et al. International clinical practice guidelines for the treatment of acute uncomplicated cystitis and pyelonephritis in women: a 2010 update by the Infectious Diseases Society of America and the European Society for Microbiology and Infectious Diseases. Clin Infect Dis. 2011;52(5):e103–20.
53. Oplinger M, Andrews CO. Nitrofurantoin contraindication in patients with a creatinine clearance below 60 mL/min: looking for the evidence. Ann Pharmacother. 2013;47(1):106–11.
54. Gupta K, Sahm DF, Mayfield D, Stamm WE. Antimicrobial resistance among uropathogens that cause community-acquired urinary tract infections in women: a nationwide analysis. Clin Infect Dis. 2001;33(1):89–94.
55. Perrotta C, Aznar M, Mejia R, Albert X, Ng CW. Oestrogens for preventing recurrent urinary tract infection in postmenopausal women. Cochrane Database of Systematic Reviews. 2008;(2).
56. Bianco L, Perrelli E, Towle V, Van Ness PH, Juthani-Mehta M. Pilot randomized controlled dosing study of cranberry capsules for reduction of bacteriuria plus pyuria in female nursing home residents. J Am Geriatr Soc. 2012;60(6):1180–1.
57. Jepson RG, Williams G, Craig JC. Cranberries for preventing urinary tract infections. Cochrane Database Syst Rev. 2012;(10):CD001321.
58. Hersh AL, Chambers HF, Maselli JH, Gonzales R. National trends in ambulatory visits and antibiotic prescribing for skin and soft-tissue infections. Arch Intern Med. 2008; 168(14):1585–91.
59. Edelsberg J, Taneja C, Zervos M, Haque N, Moore C, Reyes K, et al. Trends in US hospital admissions for skin and soft tissue infections. Emerg Infect Dis. 2009;15(9):1516–8.
60. Stevens DL, Bisno AL, Chambers HF, Dellinger EP, Goldstein EJ, Gorbach SL, et al. Practice guidelines for the diagnosis and management of skin and soft tissue infections: 2014 update by the Infectious Diseases Society of America. Clin Infect Dis. 2014;59(2):e10–52.
61. Gunderson CG, Martinello RA. A systematic review of bacteremias in cellulitis and erysipelas. J Infect. 2012;64(2):148–55.
62. Gunderson CG. Cellulitis: definition, etiology, and clinical features. Am J Med. 2011; 124(12):1113–22.
63. Whitley RJ. A 70-year-old woman with shingles: review of herpes zoster. JAMA. 2009; 302(1):73–80.
64. Cohen JI. Clinical practice: herpes zoster. N Engl J Med. 2013;369(3):255–63.
65. Oxman MN, Levin MJ, Johnson GR, Schmader KE, Straus SE, Gelb LD, et al. A vaccine to prevent herpes zoster and postherpetic neuralgia in older adults. N Engl J Med. 2005;352(22):2271–84.
66. Schmader KE, Oxman MN, Levin MJ, Johnson G, Zhang JH, Betts R, et al. Persistence of the efficacy of zoster vaccine in the shingles prevention study and the short-term persistence substudy. Clin Infect Dis. 2012;55(10):1320–8.
67. Lessa FC, Mu Y, Bamberg WM, Beldavs ZG, Dumyati GK, Dunn JR, et al. Burden of Clostridium difficile infection in the United States. N Engl J Med. 2015;372(9):825–34.
68. Henrich TJ, Krakower D, Bitton A, Yokoe DS. Clinical risk factors for severe Clostridium difficile-associated disease. Emerg Infect Dis. 2009;15(3):415–22.
69. Pawar D, Tsay R, Nelson DS, Elumalai MK, Lessa FC, Clifford McDonald L, et al. Burden of Clostridium difficile infection in long-term care facilities in Monroe County, New York. Infect Control Hosp Epidemiol. 2012;33(11):1107–12.
70. Cohen SH, Gerding DN, Johnson S, Kelly CP, Loo VG, McDonald LC, et al. Clinical practice guidelines for Clostridium difficile infection in adults: 2010 update by the society for healthcare epidemiology of America (SHEA) and the infectious diseases society of America (IDSA). Infect Control Hosp Epidemiol. 2010;31(5):431–55.
71. Koo HL, Koo DC, Musher DM, DuPont HL. Antimotility agents for the treatment of Clostridium difficile diarrhea and colitis. Clin Infect Dis. 2009;48(5):598–605.

Urinary Incontinence Among Older Adults

4

Amy Hsu, Anne M. Suskind, and Alison J. Huang

Definition, Prevalence, and Impact

Urinary incontinence (UI) is defined as involuntary leakage of urine [1]. While prevalence estimates vary with the definition used and the population studied, the overall prevalence of UI in both men and women increases with age. Worldwide, around 30–60 % of women and 3–20 % of men over the age of 60 report some UI [2]. Among older adults living in long-term care facilities, the prevalence is even higher, ranging from 43 to 77 % [3]. Although UI has not been shown to directly increase mortality in older adults, it is associated with psychological distress [4], social isolation [5], falls and fractures [6], increased caregiver burden [7], and admission to long-term care facilities [8].

Age-Related Physiological Changes in Urinary Tract Function

Physiological changes of the lower urinary tract may predispose older adults to develop UI. With aging, the muscular layer of the bladder, the detrusor muscle, tends to decrease in contraction strength, which can contribute to inadequate bladder

A. Hsu (✉)
Division of Geriatrics, Department of Medicine, San Francisco Veterans Affairs Medical Center; University of California, San Francisco, 4150 Clement Street, Box 181G, San Francisco, CA 94121, USA
e-mail: Amy.Hsu@ucsf.edu

A.M. Suskind
Department of Urology, University of California, San Francisco, 400 Parnassus, Box 0738, San Francisco, CA 94123, USA
e-mail: Anne.Suskind@ucsf.edu

A.J. Huang
Department of Medicine, University of California, San Francisco, 1545 Divisadero Street, Box 0320, San Francisco, CA 94115-1732, USA
e-mail: Alison.Huang@ucsf.edu

© Springer International Publishing Switzerland 2016
L.A. Lindquist (ed.), *New Directions in Geriatric Medicine*,
DOI 10.1007/978-3-319-28137-7_4

emptying and overflow incontinence. In older women, UI may be precipitated by the decrease in urethral closure pressure [9], which has been attributed to lower estrogen levels, decreased vascularity, decline in urethral muscle thickness [10], and decrease in density of muscle fibers [11]. There is also evidence of pelvic floor muscle denervation and decline in total collagen content associated with aging [12].

Classification of Urinary Causes of Incontinence

Determination of the primary type of UI is useful because treatment differs depending on the underlying cause. Among older adults, UI is conventionally classified as *stress, urgency, mixed, overflow,* or *functional* UI although many older adults suffer from more than one type of UI.

Stress UI Stress UI is characterized by leakage of urine associated with activities that increase intra-abdominal pressure, such as coughing, sneezing, laughing, or exercising. Stress UI develops when the urethral sphincter is unable to withstand an increase in bladder pressure. In older women, this can be due to weakness of the pelvic floor musculature from previous pregnancy, vaginal delivery, surgical scarring, decreased estrogen, or obesity. Among men, stress UI is less common due to the increased length of the urethra and the additional bladder support provided by the prostate; however, stress UI may occur after prostatectomy and transurethral surgery or as a result of radiation therapy [13, 14]. Stress UI may be unmasked or exacerbated when patients develop respiratory infections that cause more frequency of coughing or sneezing or when there is an increase in physical activity level associated with increased intra-abdominal pressure.

Urgency UI Urgency UI is characterized by strong or sudden urges to void followed by leakage of urine. The primary underlying physiologic mechanism of urgency UI is the presence of uninhibited contractions of the detrusor muscle (also known as *detrusor overactivity*), resulting in recurrent, involuntary urges to urinate. If these contractions generate enough bladder pressure to overcome the urethral sphincter mechanism, these urgency episodes may result in urine leakage [15]. Detrusor overactivity is often idiopathic in older adults and increases in prevalence with increasing age [16], which may be due to changes in release of neurotransmitters that influence bladder contraction [17]. Detrusor overactivity can also be associated with neurologic conditions that lead to decreased cortical inhibition, such as stroke, Parkinson's disease, and Alzheimer's dementia [15].

Urgency UI is often considered part of a broader syndrome known as *overactive bladder*, characterized by recurrent urges to urinate that result in daytime urinary frequency and/or nocturia [18]. Some patients with overactive bladder do not experience incontinence (i.e., "dry" overactive bladder) [19], but because the underlying pathophysiology is the same as urgency incontinence (i.e., "wet" overactive bladder) [19], approaches to management are similar regardless of whether incontinence takes place [14].

Among older adults, detrusor overactivity can coexist with impaired detrusor contractility, resulting in a condition known as "detrusor hyperactivity with impaired contractility" or *DHIC*. Detrusor hyperactivity occurs during bladder filling while impaired contractility occurs during bladder emptying, leading to urgency UI with an elevated post-void residual urine volume in the absence of bladder outlet obstruction. Patients present with leakage, hesitancy, dribbling, and frequency suggestive of overflow UI, as well as urgency UI symptoms. DHIC increases in prevalence with age [20] and is more common among older adults with cognitive deficits and restricted mobility [21]. DHIC can be difficult to diagnose and treat due to the non-specific symptoms and can also confound the diagnosis of overactive bladder [21].

Mixed UI The term "mixed UI" is used to describe the combination of urgency UI and stress UI that often coexist in older patients, particularly older female patients. Patients with mixed UI can have both stress and urgency symptoms in the same episode of incontinence or have discrete episodes of either type [22]. Because many patients with mixed UI have predominantly urgency or stress UI symptoms, eliciting the predominant type of symptom can often guide treatment. Mixed UI accounts for 10–30 % of cases of UI in men [2] and up to 50 % in women [23] and increases in prevalence with age [24].

Overflow UI Overflow UI develops when the volume of urine in the bladder exceeds bladder capacity, resulting in urine leakage. The two main mechanisms underlying overflow UI are underactive bladder and bladder outlet obstruction. *Underactive bladder* (also known as *detrusor underactivity* or *impaired detrusor contractility*) is characterized by bladder contractions of reduced strength and/or duration, resulting in impaired bladder emptying [18]. Underactive bladder can occur in the setting of acute events, such as urinary tract infection or medication use, or in the setting of chronic diseases, such as diabetes mellitus or chronic overactive bladder [25]. Older adults with underactive bladder may also have a diminished sense of when the bladder is full and are unable to contract the bladder muscles sufficiently. Prior to developing overt overflow UI, patients may develop symptoms of hesitancy, a sensation of incomplete emptying, or straining to urinate [25].

Bladder outlet obstruction can also lead to overflow UI, even in the absence of underactive bladder. Obstruction that leads to urinary retention usually causes a small amount of leakage from bladder distention. Among older men, a common cause of bladder outlet obstruction is prostate enlargement. Among older women, obstruction is rarer but may be caused by pelvic organ prolapse, urethral injury, or stricture [13, 26].

Functional UI Functional UI is defined as the loss of urine in the setting of a normal urinary system, usually due to factors such as physical and cognitive impairment or systemic illnesses. Functional UI is more common among older adults with severe disability that prevent them from recognizing the need to void or use the toilet. Some causes of functional UI are reversible and will be described in the next section [27, 28].

Distribution of Different Types of UI

Among women, the prevalence of stress UI decreases with age, from 35 % in women aged 50–59 down to 15 % in women 80 years and older. In contrast, the prevalence of urgency UI increases with age, from 9 % among women aged 50–59 up to 23 % among women 85–89 years and older [29, 30]. The prevalence of mixed UI has also been found to increase from 15 % in women 50–59 years old up to 30 % in women 80 years and older [29, 31]. Among men, urgency UI is the most common type of UI, affecting between 2.5 % and 10 % of men, while stress UI affects only 1.6–2.5 % of men [24, 32] and occurs predominantly after radical prostatectomy.

Classification of Non-urinary Causes of Incontinence

The mnemonic "DIAPPERS" has been widely used to describe common non-genitourinary tract contributors to UI in older adults [33] (Table 4.1). As many of these contributors are reversible, evaluation and treatment of these non-genitourinary tract causes are recommended before clinicians focus exclusively on potential deficits of the bladder, urethra, or pelvic floor.

Delirium Delirium is one of the most common causes of incontinence in older patients who are hospitalized or recently hospitalized [34]. A clouded sensorium can impede the recognition of both the need to void and the ability to access a toilet. When delirium is the primary cause of UI, symptoms usually clear after delirium resolves [35].

Infection Urinary tract infection can cause or contribute to urgency and incontinence [35]. Confirmation by urine culture is important to avoid overuse of antibiotics. In older women, urinary tract infection can be difficult to distinguish from asymptomatic bacteriuria, which does not warrant antibiotic treatment.

Table 4.1 Non-genitourinary causes of urinary incontinence and treatment: DIAPPERS

Cause	Treatment
Delirium	Manage delirium, commode at bedside
Infection	Confirm and treat urinary tract infection
Atrophic vaginitis or urethritis	Topical or intravaginal estrogen
Pharmaceuticals	Stop or adjust dose/schedule of medications
Psychiatric disorders	Treat depression, commode at bedside
Excessive urine production	Treat underlying condition, stop or reschedule diuretic regimen
Restricted mobility	Commode at bedside for fall prevention, physical therapy
Stool impaction	Stool dis-impaction, bowel regimen

Atrophic Vaginitis or Urethritis Among older women, atrophic urethritis may cause symptoms of dysuria or irritative voiding that can be mistaken for urinary tract infection. In a clinical context, atrophic urethritis is suggested by signs of inflammation and atrophy on pelvic exam, associated with estrogen depletion, including the presence of vaginal mucosa telangiectasia, petechiae, erosions, erythema, or friability. Diagnosis is more likely if symptoms respond to a trial of topical estrogen or other topical treatments for atrophy [35].

Pharmaceuticals Medications are common contributors of UI, particularly in older adults who are more likely to suffer from polypharmacy. Typical offending agents include medications that increase urine volume (diuretics), impair bladder contractility (anticholinergics and calcium channel blockers), exacerbate constipation (opioids), impair cognition (psychotropics, sedatives), or exacerbate prostate-related bladder outflow obstruction (alpha-agonists) [35].

Psychiatric Disorders Depression and psychomotor retardation may impede the ability or motivation of older adults to reach a toilet. Among patients with urgency UI, anxiety and psychologic stress have also been identified as possible contributors to detrusor overactivity and overactive bladder [36, 37].

Excessive Urine Output Excessive urine output can overwhelm the ability of an older adult to reach a toilet in time. Causes may include: excessive intake of fluids, diabetes mellitus (hyperglycemia), hypercalcemia, diabetes insipidus, or medications such as diuretics.

Restricted Mobility Restricted mobility can result in *functional incontinence*, whereby an older adult cannot gain access to the toilet [35, 38]. Environmental restrictions such as difficulty removing clothing may also contribute. Using a bedside commode may help with incontinence at night, with caregiver assistance to prevent falls associated with transferring.

Stool Impaction Stool impaction can be a cause of UI among hospitalized or immobilized older adults if impaction increases bladder pressure or obstructs the bladder outflow tract. Fecal incontinence may also coexist with urinary incontinence since the bowels and bladder are innervated by the same neural plexus [38].

Evaluation

Screening

Less than half of older adults with UI seek help [39], and men seek help for UI less frequently than women [40]. Therefore, systematic screening for UI has been recommended in older adults to avoid underdiagnosis of UI [41, 42]. Possible screening questions to ask include: "Do you have trouble with your bladder?" or "Do you lose urine when you do not want to?" or "Do you wear pads or adult diapers for protection?"[13]

If the patient screens positive for urinary incontinence, clinicians should attempt to establish how much the patient is bothered by the symptoms and how important UI is in the context of other health problems, in order to determine the most appropriate treatment strategy. Aside from acute reversible causes, such as urinary tract infection, treatment should be guided by patient preference, since some treatment strategies, particularly invasive ones, may be associated with their own adverse effects.

History

Once urinary incontinence is identified, assessing non-genitourinary causes of UI (using the DIAPPERS pneumonic in Table 4.1) is a reasonable starting point [13]. Chronic illnesses such as diabetes, stroke, dementia, Parkinsonism, and arthritis may be identified as contributors or causes of UI in older adults. Review of functional status, including sensory impairments and lifestyle factors such as exercise and fluid intake, may identify noninvasive modifiable factors that predispose patients to have UI [22]. A thorough review of medications is important in all older adults but can help to identify specific pharmacologic contributors to UI. Additionally, in older adults with cognitive impairment, it may be helpful to enlist caregivers to provide or supplement information on symptoms and severity [34].

After non-genitourinary factors are assessed, genitourinary causes of incontinence should be addressed, guided by the predominant type of UI, keeping in mind that a combination of factors may be contributing to the patients' symptoms. Several validated questions have been developed to help determine the type of incontinence. For stress UI, if the patient answers yes to the question, "Do you lose urine during sudden physical exertion, coughing, sneezing or lifting?" the likelihood that they have stress UI increases. If the patient answers no, stress UI is less likely to be the type of UI [22, 43]. A similar question to identify urgency incontinence is, "Do you experience such a strong and sudden urge to urinate that you leak before reaching the toilet?"[22, 43] For detrusor overactivity, asking about frequency and urgency with or without UI can help establish the diagnosis, but the absence of symptoms does not rule out the possibility of having detrusor overactivity [22, 43]. Reviewing obstetrical and gynecological history in women, such as parity, history of pelvic floor surgery, or radiation, can identify risk factors for stress UI.

After identifying the type of UI, establishing the characteristics such as duration, frequency, volume, timing, and associated factors can guide the remainder of the discussion. One way for clinicians to establish severity is to ask about the number of pads used, type of pad, frequency of pad changing, and degree of pad saturation as indicators of the severity of UI symptoms [44]. Voiding diaries may be a more accurate way of recalling symptom frequency and severity. Eliciting from the patient his or her most bothersome symptoms and their impact on daily life can ensure a patient-centered discussion [13].

Voiding Diary

For patients who have difficulty recalling and characterizing their voiding and incontinence episodes, a daily voiding or bladder diary can be useful for documenting and classifying symptoms as well as monitoring response to therapies. Patients may be instructed to record their oral fluid intake volume and type, timing of episodes of urinary leakage and voids into the toilet, volume of urine lost per voiding episode, and precipitators of incontinence, as well as relationship to activities and sleep. Recording for 3–7 days is usually sufficient to determine the general type of symptoms and may prevent diary fatigue [44]. An example of a daily bladder diary can be found on the National Kidney and Urologic Diseases Information Clearing House website (http://kidney.niddk.nih.gov/Kudiseases/pubs/diary/index.aspx).

Questionnaires

A variety of validated questionnaires have been developed to detect and distinguish between clinical types of UI. The 3 Incontinence Questions (3IQ) is a three-item questionnaire that was validated in 301 community-dwelling, ambulatory women up to age 94 and can be used to diagnose urgency and stress UI in women [45]. Using subspecialty evaluation as the gold standard, the questionnaire has a sensitivity of 0.75 and specificity of 0.77 for classifying urgency UI and a sensitivity of 0.86 and specificity of 0.60 for classifying stress UI.

The Michigan Incontinence Symptom Index (M-ISI) is a ten-item questionnaire that can be used in both men and women to distinguish between stress UI, urgency UI, and mixed UI as well as to gauge severity and bother from UI [46]. This index was validated in women up to age 88. Higher scores represent greater symptoms and bother. Screening cutoffs have been established for each subtype of UI in the questionnaire: a score of ≥ 3 (questions 1–3) is positive for clinically significant stress UI, a score of ≥ 5 (questions 4–6) is positive for clinically significant urgency UI, and a score of ≥ 7 screens positive for the entire questionnaire [47]. A minimum change of 4 points correspond to a beneficial change in UI for patients [46].

In men, the American Urological Association Symptom Index (AUA-SI) can identify lower urinary tract symptoms associated bladder outlet obstruction [26], which can help guide further evaluation and treatment, although this index does not specifically address urinary incontinence.

Physical Exam

Physical examination should be tailored to the specific symptoms reported by the patient. A patient at risk for constipation and fecal impaction may need a rectal examination to identify and treat fecal impaction and assess sphincter tone and perineal sensation [14, 38]. For patients reporting possible overflow UI symptoms, an abdominal examination can identify severe bladder distention but is insensitive for ruling out elevated post-void residual urine volume. Because of the high prevalence of cognitive dysfunction and/or functional impairment among older adults, assessing the severity of these conditions may help determine whether they are contributing to UI. Among older men reporting possible obstructive urinary symptoms, a prostate examination to identify prostate enlargement may be indicated.

In older women, a pelvic examination may help confirm a diagnosis of stress UI, identify significant pelvic prolapse, detect possibly malignant masses, or reveal signs of inflammation suggesting atrophic vaginitis as contributors to UI symptoms [14]. Pelvic examination may be more uncomfortable in older women due to pain or limitations in mobility, however, and thus, it may be appropriate to modify or tailor the exam to minimize discomfort in older patients. A bimanual examination may be sufficient to detect abnormalities such as pelvic prolapse that is visible without the use of a speculum. If a speculum examination is needed, clinicians can use an ultra-narrow speculum and additional lubricant in women with possible vulvovaginal atrophy. Topical lidocaine can also be applied prior to the speculum and bimanual examination to minimize discomfort. Patients with limited mobility or joint pain may be more comfortable in alternative positions than lithotomy, such as the lateral position (lying on one side with hips and knees flexed) or the V position (supine, hips abducted, knees extended) [48].

The supine empty bladder stress test (SEBST) can help diagnose severe stress UI in women [49]. The test is performed after the patient voids. While in a supine position, the patient is instructed to cough or Valsalva. Any leakage from the urethral meatus during this maneuver provides positive evidence of stress UI. The SEBST has been shown to correlate with objective measures of UI severity, such as patient-reported UI frequency, as well as response to questionnaires on the impact of UI [49].

Tests/Labs

For all older patients with urgency, a urinalysis should be performed to assess for hematuria, pyuria, or glucosuria. If there is hematuria, defined as more than three red blood cells per high-powered field on microscopy, and this hematuria persists upon repeat testing, further urologic investigation is warranted [38]. Obtaining a sample via straight catheterization may be necessary if bacterial contamination is a concern in older women who may have difficulty obtaining a clean catch sample.

For older patients with possible overflow incontinence, measurement of post-void residual (PVR) urine volume, either by ultrasound or bladder catheterization, may be indicated to evaluate for urinary retention. Because PVR measurements can be difficult to obtain in a primary care setting, assessments should be focused on patients at increased risk for bladder outlet obstruction or incomplete bladder emptying. Among older women, this may include those with pelvic organ prolapse, diabetes mellitus with neurologic sequelae, and stroke or those taking medications that may promote urinary retention [50]. In older men with mild to moderate symptoms, routine PVR testing is not required unless bladder outlet obstruction is suspected [51].

Complicating the interpretation of PVR is that the range of normal PVR is not standardized, and there is evidence that elevated PVR does not always correlate with urinary symptoms in older women [52]. Conventionally, a PVR of greater than 200 mL is considered elevated, although studies suggest that a high proportion of individuals with a single PVR in this range go on to have normal PVR upon repeat assessment [52]. In patients with PVR persistently over 300 mL, clinicians may also consider testing serum creatinine to assess for renal failure, which is associated with chronically elevated PVR [53].

Treatment

Before starting treatment, clinicians should discuss patients' treatment priorities and establish measurable goals to ensure that the treatment plan is consistent with patients' wishes [53]. Patients may have goals other than simply decreasing the frequency or volume of leakage, such as taking part in social activities or decreasing caregiver burden [54]. It is also important to set realistic expectations that cure from UI may not be attainable, particularly if patients are suffering from frequent or severe UI at baseline.

General Treatments

Lifestyle Modification

Lifestyle modifications can be used alone or in addition to clinical treatments to manage UI. These modifications include reducing caffeine intake, changing the timing of oral fluid intake, and weight loss (among patients who are overweight or obese) [54]. Large studies in men [32] and women [55, 56] have shown that consumption of caffeine equivalent to 2–4 cups of coffee per day is associated with UI symptoms. If caffeine-containing beverages comprise a large portion of daily fluid intake, patients may benefit from reduction in intake to fewer than two cups, although this strategy has not been evaluated in controlled interventional studies. Overall oral fluid intake likely contributes little to the pathogenesis of UI [57], and older adults should consume at least 30 ml/kg of fluids per day to keep up with metabolic losses [58]. For older adults who have trouble reaching a bathroom or have nighttime UI, however, restricting fluids before going to bed may help control symptoms.

Weight loss has also been shown to improve UI in overweight and obese women [59] presumably because decrease abdominal weight leads to lower intra-bladder pressure. This includes not only surgical weight loss through bariatric procedures [60] but also weight loss achieved through diet and exercise interventions [61]. Studies of the effects of weight loss on UI have not tended to include frail older adults, however, in whom weight loss can be a poor prognostic sign, particularly if weight loss takes the form of muscle mass rather than fat mass.

Protective Garments and Pads

Older adults, particularly those who live in long-term care facilities or who are dependent on caregivers for activities of daily living, may prefer the use of pads or protective undergarments to manage UI [62, 63]. From the few trials that assessed patient preference, disposable pull-ups are preferred by women but are the most expensive, while diapers were the most cost-effective for men [64]. If pads or diapers are preferred, gentle cleansing with a disposable soft cloth and use of a skin protectant can prevent skin breakdown [65].

Behavioral Interventions

After non-urinary causes of incontinence (i.e., DIAPPERS) have been addressed and applicable lifestyle modifications implemented, behavioral interventions are the mainstay of treatment, especially among frail older adults [66]. These interventions include: prompted voiding, bladder retraining, timed voiding, and combined toileting and exercise therapy [66]. *Prompted voiding* involves prompting the patient to toilet with contingent social approval to increase patient requests for toileting or self-initiated toileting [66]. Prompted voiding can decrease UI episodes for the short term [67] in nursing home residents or home-care clients who are able to state their name, transfer with assistance of one person, and have caregivers who are willing to assist [68]. *Bladder retraining* involves identifying a patient's voiding habits and then setting up a toileting schedule to preempt UI episodes [69]. Trials on habit retraining in older adults with physical and/or cognitive impairment have found that the protocols were time intensive for caregivers to follow and the benefits were unclear [69]. A less intensive intervention is *timed voiding*, which aims to schedule a patient's voiding times at fixed intervals. Two trials on timed voiding combined with other interventions showed that timed voiding may decrease nighttime UI [70]. *Combined toileting and exercise therapy* which incorporates strengthening exercises in addition to toileting routines has been shown to reduce the percentage of wet checks showing UI by 20 % [71] but may require trained staff [72].

Pelvic Floor Muscle Training

Pelvic floor muscle training (PFMT or Kegel exercises) is a key component of noninvasive UI treatment and has been shown to be effective for urgency UI, stress UI, and mixed UI [54]. These exercises involve repeated voluntary pelvic floor muscle contractions [73] to increase muscle strength, endurance, and coordination [58]. Efficacy depends on whether patients are able to identify and isolate the correct muscles, as well as adherence to frequent and sustained practice [54]. Therefore, supervised PFMT programs may be more effective than self-directed programs [58] although data from randomized-controlled trials provide limited data for comparison [74]. Among female patients with stress UI, the NNT (number needed to treat) of PFMT compared to no active treatment to achieve continence is 3 [75]. PFMT has been shown to decrease urgency UI by an average of 1.2 episodes per day and mixed UI by 0.7 episodes per day, compared with 0.9 episodes for stress UI [76].

Other interventions have been used to enhance PFMT, including biofeedback, where a health professional or a vaginal device can let the patient know how well the pelvic floor muscles are activated and can potentially enhance the results of PFMT, but randomized-control trials among women were biased in that women who received biofeedback spent more time in the clinical setting compared to women in the control groups [77]. Vaginal cones, which are inserted into the vagina and prevented from slipping out with active pelvic floor muscle contractions, can also be used to provide progressive muscular load with PFMT [78]. Pelvic floor electrical stimulation with surface electrodes placed in the vaginal can also be added to PFMT [39]. PFMT is particularly effective in improving and curing stress UI but can be used in all subtypes of UI [79]. Trials of PFMT have ranged in duration from 4 weeks to 6 months [80]. Telling patients to anticipate that a course of PFMT can be 6–10 weeks, 3–5 days per week, and may take even longer to see clinical changes can help set expectations for the amount of time and effort required to see progress.

In men, there is insufficient evidence to show benefit from PFMT for urinary incontinence after prostate surgery [81]. However, electrical stimulation with surface electrode devices may improve symptoms in the short term (6 months) when used with PFMT [82].

Urgency UI Specific Treatments

Urge suppression and *bladder training* are two behavioral techniques specifically designed to address urgency incontinence. Urge suppression employs a combination of distraction and relaxation techniques to divert attention away from the sensation of urgency while pelvic floor muscle exercises are used to suppress detrusor contractions. Upon experiencing an urge to urinate, patients are taught to avoid rushing to the toilet but instead to remain still, take slow deep breaths, purposefully activate their pelvic floor muscles, and wait for the urge to pass [54]. Urge suppression is often combined with bladder training techniques that schedule voiding at increasingly extended intervals to decrease voiding frequency, increase bladder capacity, and restore normal bladder function [54, 75]. Among women, the NNT to improve UI for bladder training compared to no active treatment is 2 [75]. Bladder training can be combined with PFMT, though trials have not shown additional benefit [83].

If behavioral treatment methods are not successful in controlling urgency UI, *antimuscarinic medications* may be effective in improving the frequency of UI episodes. These medications should be started at the lowest dose available after checking for drug interactions with the patient's existing medications [54]. Anti-muscarinic agents decrease detrusor contraction by blocking acetylcholine stimulation of muscarinic receptors [84]. In systematic reviews of effects in female patients, the different anti-muscarinic agents provide similar improvement in UI symptoms when compared to placebo, with the number needed to treat (to achieve continence) ranging from 6 to 12 [75] (Table 4.2). When looking only at studies that include older adults, the average benefit was a reduction of fewer than one leakage episode per 24 h [88].

Table 4.2 Anti-muscarinic agents

Anti-muscarinic agents for urgency UI	Dose	NNT[a] (compared to placebo, to achieve continence)	Dose adjustments	Side effects: (common for all agents: dry mouth, constipation, dyspepsia, headaches, dizziness, decrease gastrointestinal motility)[c]	NNH[a] (compared to placebo, for side effects)
Darifenacin	7.5–15 mg daily	9[b]	Max dose 7.5 mg daily for hepatic impairment	Lower rate of CNS effects in older adults[c]	
Fesoterodine	4–8 mg daily	8	Max dose 4 mg if CrCl <30		
Oxybutynin	IR: 2.5 mg 2–3 times daily	9		Insomnia, adverse skin reaction to transdermal route; fewer reported side effects with transdermal route	
	XL: 5–30 mg daily				
	Patch: one patch twice per week				
Solifenacin	5–10 mg daily	9	Max dose 5 mg daily for CrCl <30 or hepatic impairment	QT prolongation[d]	6
Tolterodine	IR: 1–2 mg twice daily	12	Max dose 1 mg twice daily (IR) and 2 mg daily (ER) for CrCl <30; avoid use in hepatic impairment	QT prolongation[d], hallucinations	12
	ER: 2–4 mg daily				
Tropsium	20 mg daily	9	Max dose 20 mg daily for CrCl <30; avoid use with hepatic impairment	Dizziness; fewer cognitive side effects (should not cross blood brain barrier)[d]	8
Mirabegron	25–50 mg		Max dose 25 mg daily if CrCl <30; avoid use with hepatic impairment	Monitor heart rate and blood pressure	

NNH number needed to harm

[a]Qaseem et al. [75]

[b]Outcome was improvement in UI rather than achieve continence

[c]Macdiarmid [85], Chughtai et al. [86]

[d]Hesch [87]

Common side effects of anti-muscarinic medications include dry mouth, constipation, dyspepsia, headaches, and dizziness. More than half of patients stop taking anti-muscarinic medications after 1 year of treatment [89]. The incidence for acute urinary retention while taking an anti-muscarinic agent increases with age and is up to 6.9/1000 person-years among men aged 88–84 years [90]. Furthermore, many trials of anti-muscarinic medications have excluded men with elevated post-void residual volumes at baseline, therefore underestimating the overall risk [91]. As a result, patients may require monitoring of post-void residual urine volumes or symptoms of urinary retention for the first 30 days after starting the medication [90]. An additional concern is the effect of anti-muscarinic agents on cognition in older adults. Worsening memory and recall after treatment with extended-release oxybutynin has been reported [92]. Higher cumulative doses of anticholinergic agents, including anti-muscarinic agents, over a 10-year period were found to increase the risk of dementia [93]. Additionally, anti-muscarinic agents are contraindicated in patients with known urinary or gastric retention and uncontrolled angle-closure glaucoma [87].

A new class of medications, *beta-3-adrenoceptor agonists*, became available in 2012 to treat urgency UI and overactive bladder and provide a potential alternative for patients wishing to avoid the side effects of anti-muscarinic agents. Mirabegron is currently the only available agent in this class, with an NNT (to achieve continence) of 12 [75]. In phase 2 and 3 studies, about 550 patients were 75 and older (representing 10 % of the patients) and no difference in safety or efficacy was observed between those 65 years and older versus those younger than 65 [94]. The most frequent adverse events leading to discontinuation were nausea, headache, hypertension, diarrhea, constipation, dizziness, and tachycardia [94]. In the post-marketing phase, urinary retention has also been reported, leading to the Food and Drug Administration (FDA) to caution use in patients with bladder outlet obstruction [94]. Data are currently limited to indicate the efficacy and safety of mirabegron in combination with anti-muscarinic agents.

In men with urgency UI and bladder outlet obstruction, *alpha-blockers* may be better tolerated than anti-muscarinic agents but can cause orthostatic hypotension and dizziness. If UI symptoms persist after appropriate titration of an alpha-blocker, an anti-muscarinic agent can be added [95]. Checking a post-void residual urine volume before initiation may be appropriate in patients at risk for retention [26]. The combined side effects from both an anti-muscarinic agent and alpha-blocker can be concerning for frail older adults at risk for falls and altered mental status.

Stress UI Specific Treatments

Timed pelvic muscle contraction is a maneuver performed prior to activities or motions that cause stress-type leakage and has been shown to be helpful for women with mild to moderate stress UI [96]. The maneuver involves increasing pelvic muscle strength and using pelvic muscles to consciously occlude the urethra during or prior to activities that cause leakage, such as before sneezing or coughing [54].

Pessaries are intravaginal devices that are inserted under the urethra to increase urethral support and decrease stress UI in women with pelvic organ prolapse [97]. Pessaries require proper fitting for comfort and effectiveness [98] but can be removed, cleaned, and reinserted in a clinic every 4–6 weeks for women who may have difficulty inserting them at home [54]. Pessaries have been shown to improve UI compared with no treatment and may potentially be more effective when combined with PFMT [99]. Although pessaries are associated with a risk of vaginal tissue erosion or discharge, such events are rare with proper use [98].

Nonsystemic estrogen has shown some efficacy compared to placebo for the treatment of stress UI in women. Vaginal estrogen can be given in the form of cream, ovules, or tablets, although a concomitant progestin may be necessary to prevent development of endometrial hyperplasia if full-dose vaginal estrogen is used [100]. Although systemic absorption is much lower than with oral or transdermal estrogen, the use of vaginal estrogen is still relatively contraindicated in patients with a history of breast cancer or other estrogen-associated cancers [101]. Side effects of vaginal estrogen include vaginal discharge, uterine bleeding, breast pain, and perineal pain. Systemic transdermal estrogen patches are associated with worsening of UI symptoms and, like oral estrogen preparations, should not be used to treat UI [75]. The NNT of vaginal estrogen tablets and vaginal ovules compared to placebo for improving continence is 5 [75].

Although systemic pharmacological treatments such as *alpha-adrenergic agonists* and the serotonin-reuptake inhibitor duloxetine have been explored for stress UI, they are not currently approved for this indication in the USA, due to studies suggesting insufficient efficacy in comparison to adverse effects [73, 98].

When to Refer to a Specialist

Referral to a specialist is appropriate for patients who have a complicated initial presentation. In women, this includes UI symptoms with pain, hematuria, recurrent infections, significant pelvic organ prolapse, history of pelvic irradiation or surgery, or suspected fistula. In men, suspected or proven poor bladder emptying is an additional reason for referral [102].

Among patients with an uncomplicated initial presentation, referral to a specialist may be indicated after a trial of behavioral therapy, PFMT, and one or more medications (in the case of urgency-type UI) and if the patient continues to be sufficiently bothered by UI symptoms such that he or she would consider invasive treatment. The following are treatment options that may be helpful to discuss with patients to assess whether referral to a specialist would be helpful:

Specialist Urgency UI Treatments

Percutaneous tibial nerve stimulation (*PTNS*) involves insertion of a fine needle into the skin of the lower extremity, near the medial malleolus, in order to deliver an adjustable electoral pulse to the sacral plexus via the tibial nerve (i.e., neuromodulation). Treatment lasts for 30 min at a time and is typically performed once a week for 12 weeks in an outpatient setting [54] and can be followed by maintenance treatment [103].

Sacral neuromodulation is a more invasive neuromodulation treatment strategy involving surgical placement of electrodes through the S3 nerve foramen. If the treatment is successful after a short trial period, a permanent lead and implantable pulse generator can be inserted surgically [103]. Outcomes in older adults (over age 55) have shown at least 50 % reduction in UI symptoms, but the reported cure rate of 17 % was lower in comparison to younger patients [104].

Botulinum toxin injection via cystoscopy into the detrusor muscle [54] is FDA approved for the treatment of overactive bladder refractory to more conservative treatment [103], but it has not been tested rigorously in older adults [54]. The risk of botulinum injection includes temporary urinary retention (6 %) that may require self-catheterization until the effects of the toxin have worn off and urinary tract infections associated with incomplete emptying [103].

Specialist Stress UI Treatments

Periurethral injection is a minimally invasive option for both male and female patients with stress UI that can be performed in the office setting or in the operating room. Bulking agents are injected into the urethral submucosa to increase resistance of the urethral outlet [105, 106]. In uncontrolled studies, the injections have been reported to have good short-term cure rates in women, 70 % at 1 year and 50 % at 3 years [107], and the injections can be repeated [106]. Potential complications from the procedures include urinary retention and dysuria [108].

Surgical treatment can be an option for patients with stress UI who have not improved with conservative treatment. Commonly performed surgical procedures include sling and artificial sphincter placement [106, 109]. *Slings* are pieces of synthetic mesh or tissue that are surgically placed under the urethra in order to reinforce the urethral sphincter [106]. In women, slings can be placed transvaginally via minimally invasive or single-incision surgery. Reported cure rates range from 77 to 96 % among older women [73]. In men, slings can be placed in those with post-prostatectomy stress UI who have not improved with noninvasive treatment [105].

Artificial urinary sphincters (AUS) are devices consisting of a cuff around the urethra, a fluid reservoir that fills the cuff, and an activation pump. The cuff is activated to compress the urethra to withstand increased bladder pressure associated with activities and can be deactivated to allow voiding [110]. Artificial urinary sphincter placement is primarily indicated in men who have intrinsic sphincter deficiency, commonly caused by prostatectomy, transurethral resection of the prostate, or pelvic surgery [111]. The device can also be used to treat women with stress UI after radical pelvic surgery.

Key Points
1. Urinary incontinence is common among older adults in both community and institutional settings. With age, urgency incontinence increases in prevalence.
2. Less than half of older adults with urinary incontinence bring up this problem to their provider. Consider screening for urinary incontinence.
3. Evaluating non-urinary causes (DIAPPERS) of urinary incontinence first may improve symptoms without resorting to medications or procedures.
4. Identifying the primary type of urinary incontinence (urgency, stress, mixed, overflow, functional) will direct treatment.
5. Voiding diaries are helpful for assessing urinary incontinence at baseline and for following and assessing treatment efficacy.
6. Before starting treatment, establish treatment goals and health priorities with the patient, and set realistic expectations.
7. In older adults, start with the lifestyle modifications, behavioral treatments, and pelvic floor muscle training. Some older adults may also prefer protective garments to manage their urinary incontinence.
8. Anti-muscarinic agents have many side effects and should be started only after behavioral treatments and pelvic floor muscle training have not been successful and the patient remains significantly bothered by urinary incontinence. Anti-muscarinic agents should be started at a low dose, and the patient should be monitored closely.
9. In men with urgency urinary incontinence and bladder outlet obstruction, if an anti-muscarinic agent will be added to an alpha-blocker, consider checking a post-void residual, and monitor for signs of urinary retention in the first 30 days of dual therapy.
10. Referral to a specialist is appropriate after behavioral treatments, pelvic muscle floor therapy, and at least one medication has been tried and the patient remains significantly bothered by urinary incontinence. Referral is also appropriate initially if the presentation is complicated (pain, hematuria, or poor bladder emptying).

References

1. Lakhan P, Jones M, Wilson A, Courtney M, Hirdes J, Gray LC. A prospective cohort study of geriatric syndromes among older medical patients admitted to acute care hospitals. J Am Geriatr Soc. 2011;59(11):2001–8.
2. Buckley BS, Lapitan MC, Epidemiology Committee of the Fourth International Consultation on Incontinence, Paris, 2008. Prevalence of urinary incontinence in men, women, and children–current evidence: findings of the fourth international consultation on incontinence. Urology. 2010;76(2):265–70.
3. Offermans MP, Du Moulin MF, Hamers JP, Dassen T, Halfens RJ. Prevalence of urinary incontinence and associated risk factors in nursing home residents: a systematic review. Neurourol Urodyn. 2009;28(4):288–94.
4. Bogner HR, Gallo JJ, Sammel MD, Ford DE, Armenian HK, Eaton WW. Urinary incontinence and psychological distress in community-dwelling older adults. J Am Geriatr Soc. 2002;50(3):489–95.

5. Fultz NH, Fisher GG, Jenkins KR. Does urinary incontinence affect middle-aged and older women's time use and activity patterns? Obstet Gynecol. 2004;104(6):1327–34.
6. Brown JS, Vittinghoff E, Wyman JF, et al. Urinary incontinence: does it increase risk for falls and fractures? Study of Osteoporotic Fractures Research Group. J Am Geriatr Soc. 2000;48(7):721–5.
7. Langa KM, Fultz NH, Saint S, Kabeto MU, Herzog AR. Informal caregiving time and costs for urinary incontinence in older individuals in the United States. J Am Geriatr Soc. 2002;50(4):733–7.
8. Thom DH, Haan MN, Van Den Eeden SK. Medically recognized urinary incontinence and risks of hospitalization, nursing home admission and mortality. Age Ageing. 1997;26(5):367–74.
9. Trowbridge ER, Wei JT, Fenner DE, Ashton-Miller JA, Delancey JO. Effects of aging on lower urinary tract and pelvic floor function in nulliparous women. Obstet Gynecol. 2007;109(3):715–20.
10. Perucchini D, DeLancey JO, Ashton-Miller JA, Galecki A, Schaer GN. Age effects on urethral striated muscle. II. Anatomic location of muscle loss. Am J Obstet Gynecol. 2002;186(3):356–60.
11. Perucchini D, DeLancey JO, Ashton-Miller JA, Peschers U, Kataria T. Age effects on urethral striated muscle. I. Changes in number and diameter of striated muscle fibers in the ventral urethra. Am J Obstet Gynecol. 2002;186(3):351–5.
12. Tinelli A, Malvasi A, Rahimi S, et al. Age-related pelvic floor modifications and prolapse risk factors in postmenopausal women. Menopause. 2010;17(1):204–12.
13. Gibbs CF, Johnson 2nd TM, Ouslander JG. Office management of geriatric urinary incontinence. Am J Med. 2007;120(3):211–20.
14. Johnson TM, Ouslander JG. Incontinence. In: Halter JB, Ouslander JG, Tinetti ME, Studenski S, High KP, Asthana S, editors. Hazzard's geriatric medicine and gerontology, 6e. 6th ed. New York: McGraw-Hill; 2009.
15. Williams M, Pannill F. Urinary incontinence in the elderly. Ann Intern Med. 1982;97:895–907.
16. Nygaard I. Clinical practice. Idiopathic urgency urinary incontinence. N Engl J Med. 2010;363(12):1156–62.
17. Yoshida M, Miyamae K, Iwashita H, Otani M, Inadome A. Management of detrusor dysfunction in the elderly: changes in acetylcholine and adenosine triphosphate release during aging. Urology. 2004;63(3 Suppl 1):17–23.
18. Abrams P, Cardozo L, Fall M, et al. The standardisation of terminology in lower urinary tract function: report from the standardisation sub-committee of the International Continence Society. Urology. 2003;61(1):37–49.
19. Griebling TL. Overactive bladder in elderly men: epidemiology, evaluation, clinical effects, and management. Curr Urol Rep. 2013;14(5):418–25.
20. Resnick NM, Yalla SV. Detrusor hyperactivity with impaired contractile function. An unrecognized but common cause of incontinence in elderly patients. JAMA. 1987;257(22):3076–81.
21. Taylor 3rd JA, Kuchel GA. Detrusor underactivity: clinical features and pathogenesis of an underdiagnosed geriatric condition. J Am Geriatr Soc. 2006;54(12):1920–32.
22. Holroyd-Leduc JM, Tannenbaum C, Thorpe KE, Straus SE. What type of urinary incontinence does this woman have? JAMA. 2008;299(12):1446–56.
23. Melville JL, Katon W, Delaney K, Newton K. Urinary incontinence in US women: a population-based study. Arch Intern Med. 2005;165(5):537–42.
24. Irwin DE, Milsom I, Hunskaar S, et al. Population-based survey of urinary incontinence, overactive bladder, and other lower urinary tract symptoms in five countries: results of the EPIC study. Eur Urol. 2006;50(6):1306–14. discussion 1314-5.
25. Miyazato M, Yoshimura N, Chancellor MB. The other bladder syndrome: underactive bladder. Rev Urol. 2013;15(1):11–22.
26. McVary KT, Roehrborn CG, Avins AL, et al. American Urological Association Guideline: Management of Benign Prostatic Hyperplasia (BPH). American Urological Association

Education and Research, Inc. 2010. Retrieved from. http://www.auanet.org/education/guide-lines/benign-prostatic-hyperplasia.cfm. Accessed 15 Feb 2016.

27. Gammack JK. Urinary incontinence. In: Williams BA, Chang A, Ahalt C, et al., editors. Current diagnosis & treatment: geriatrics, 2e. New York: McGraw-Hill Education; 2014.

28. Tarnay CM. Chapter 42. Urinary incontinence & pelvic floor disorders. In: DeCherney AH, Nathan L, Laufer N, Roman AS, editors. CURRENT diagnosis & treatment: obstetrics & gynecology, 11e. New York: The McGraw-Hill Companies; 2013.

29. Minassian VA, Stewart WF, Wood GC. Urinary incontinence in women: variation in preva-lence estimates and risk factors. Obstet Gynecol. 2008;111(2 Pt 1):324–31.

30. Hannestad YS, Rortveit G, Sandvik H, Hunskaar S, Norwegian EPINCONT study. Epidemiology of Incontinence in the County of Nord-Trondelag. A community-based epide-miological survey of female urinary incontinence: the Norwegian EPINCONT study. Epidemiology of Incontinence in the County of Nord-Trondelag. J Clin Epidemiol. 2000;53(11):1150–7.

31. Jeong SJ, Kim HJ, Lee YJ, et al. Prevalence and clinical features of detrusor underactivity among elderly with lower urinary tract symptoms: a comparison between men and women. Korean J Urol. 2012;53(5):342–8.

32. Davis NJ, Vaughan CP, Johnson 2nd TM, et al. Caffeine intake and its association with uri-nary incontinence in United States men: results from National Health and Nutrition Examination Surveys 2005-2006 and 2007-2008. J Urol. 2013;189(6):2170–4.

33. Resnick NM. Urinary incontinence in the elderly. Med Grand Rounds. 1984;3:281–90.

34. DuBeau CE. Beyond the bladder: management of urinary incontinence in older women. Clin Obstet Gynecol. 2007;50(3):720–34.

35. Harper GM, Johnston CB, Landefeld CS. Geriatric disorders. In: Papadakis MA, McPhee SJ, Rabow MW, editors. Current medical diagnosis & treatment 2015. New York: McGraw-Hill Education; 2014.

36. Perry S, McGrother CW, Turner K, Leicestershire MRC Incontinence Study Group. An investigation of the relationship between anxiety and depression and urge incontinence in women: development of a psychological model. Br J Health Psychol. 2006;11(Pt 3):463–82.

37. Lim JR, Bak CW, Lee JB. Comparison of anxiety between patients with mixed incontinence and those with stress urinary incontinence. Scand J Urol Nephrol. 2007;41(5):403–6.

38. American Urological Association. Urinary incontinence medical student curriculum. 2012. Retrieved from http://www.auanet.org/education/urinary-incontinence.cfm. Accessed 15 Feb 2016.

39. Goode PS, Burgio KL, Richter HE, Markland AD. Incontinence in older women. JAMA. 2010;303(21):2172–81.

40. Harris SS, Link CL, Tennstedt SL, Kusek JW, McKinlay JB. Care seeking and treatment for urinary incontinence in a diverse population. J Urol. 2007;177(2):680–4.

41. Agency for Healthcare Research and Quality (AHRQ). Management of urinary incontinence in older adults: the percentage of Medicare members 65 years of age and older who reported having urine leakage in the past six months and who discussed their urinary leakage prob-lem with a health care provider. National Quality Measures Clearinghouse Measure Summary. 2015. Retrieved from https://www.qualitymeasures.ahrq.gov/content.aspx?id=48666. Accessed 15 Feb 2016.

42. National Committee for Quality Assurance. Specifications for the medicare health outcomes survey volume 6. Healthcare Effectiveness Data and Information Set (HEDIS). 2015; 29–31. Retrieved from http://www.hosonline.org/globalassets/hos-online/publications/hos_hedis_volume6_2015.pdf. Accessed 15 Feb 2016.

43. McGee S. Simplifying likelihood ratios. J Gen Intern Med. 2002;17(8):646–9.

44. Hoffman BL, Schorge JO, Schaffer JI, et al. Chapter 23. Urinary incontinence. In: Williams gynecology, 2e. New York: The McGraw-Hill Companies; 2012.

45. Brown JS, Bradley CS, Subak LL, et al. The sensitivity and specificity of a simple test to distinguish between urge and stress urinary incontinence. Ann Intern Med. 2006;144(10):715–23.

46. Suskind AM, Dunn RL, Morgan DM, DeLancey JO, McGuire EJ, Wei JT. The Michigan Incontinence Symptom Index (M-ISI): a clinical measure for type, severity, and bother related to urinary incontinence. Neurourol Urodyn. 2014;33(7):1128–34.
47. Suskind AM, Dunn RL, Morgan DM, DeLancey JO, Rew KT, Wei JT. A screening tool for clinically relevant urinary incontinence. Neurourol Urodyn. 2015;34(4):332–5.
48. Bates CK, Carroll N, Potter J. The challenging pelvic examination. J Gen Intern Med. 2011;26(6):651–7.
49. Nager CW, Kraus SR, Kenton K, et al. Urodynamics, the supine empty bladder stress test, and incontinence severity. Neurourol Urodyn. 2010;29(7):1306–11.
50. Abrams P, Andersson KE, Birder L, et al. In: Recommendation of the international scientific committee: evaluation and treatment of urinary incontinence, pelvic organ prolapse and faecal incontinence. 5th-9th July 2008, 2009. 1767–1820
51. Burden H, Warren K, Abrams P. Diagnosis of male incontinence. Curr Opin Urol. 2013;23(6):509–14.
52. Huang AJ, Brown JS, Boyko EJ, et al. Clinical significance of postvoid residual volume in older ambulatory women. J Am Geriatr Soc. 2011;59(8):1452–8.
53. Fung CH, Spencer B, Eslami M, Crandall C. Quality indicators for the screening and care of urinary incontinence in vulnerable elders. J Am Geriatr Soc. 2007;55 Suppl 2:S443–9.
54. Goode PS, Burgio KL, Locher JL, et al. Effect of behavioral training with or without pelvic floor electrical stimulation on stress incontinence in women: a randomized controlled trial. JAMA. 2003;290(3):345–52.
55. Jura YH, Townsend MK, Curhan GC, Resnick NM, Grodstein F. Caffeine intake, and the risk of stress, urgency and mixed urinary incontinence. J Urol. 2011;185(5):1775–80.
56. Gleason JL, Richter HE, Redden DT, Goode PS, Burgio KL, Markland AD. Caffeine and urinary incontinence in US women. Int Urogynecol J. 2013;24(2):295–302.
57. Hay-Smith J, Berghmans B, Burgio K, et al. Adult conservative management. In: Proceedings of the 4th international consultation on incontinence. 2009. 1025–1120
58. Dumoulin C, Hunter KF, Moore K, et al. Conservative management for female urinary incontinence and pelvic organ prolapse review 2013: summary of the 5th international consultation on incontinence. Neurourol Urodyn. 2014. doi:10.1002/nau.22677.
59. Wing RR, Creasman JM, West DS, et al. Improving urinary incontinence in overweight and obese women through modest weight loss. Obstet Gynecol. 2010;116(2 Pt 1):284–92.
60. Subak LL, King WC, Belle SH, et al. Urinary incontinence before and after bariatric surgery. JAMA Intern Med. 2015;175:1378–87.
61. Subak LL, Wing R, West DS, et al. Weight loss to treat urinary incontinence in overweight and obese women. N Engl J Med. 2009;360(5):481–90.
62. Johnson TM, Ouslander JG, Uman GC, Schnelle JF. Urinary incontinence treatment preferences in long-term care. J Am Geriatr Soc. 2001;49(6):710–8.
63. Pfisterer MH, Johnson 2nd TM, Jenetzky E, Hauer K, Oster P. Geriatric patients' preferences for treatment of urinary incontinence: a study of hospitalized, cognitively competent adults aged 80 and older. J Am Geriatr Soc. 2007;55(12):2016–22.
64. Fader M, Cottenden AM, Getliffe K. Absorbent products for moderate-heavy urinary and/or faecal incontinence in women and men. Cochrane Database Syst Rev. 2008;4:CD007408. doi:10.1002/14651858.CD007408.
65. Gray M. Incontinence-related skin damage: essential knowledge. Ostomy Wound Manage. 2007;53(12):28–32.
66. Wagg A, Gibson W, Ostaszkiewicz J, et al. Urinary incontinence in frail elderly persons: report from the 5th international consultation on incontinence. Neurourol Urodyn. 2014;34:398–406.
67. Eustice S, Roe B, Patterson J. Prompted voiding for the management of urinary incontinence in adults. Cochrane Database Syst Rev.2000;(2): CD002113.
68. DuBeau CE, Kuchel GA, Johnson 2nd T, Palmer MH, Wagg A. Incontinence in the frail elderly: report from the 4th international consultation on incontinence. Neurourol Urodyn. 2010;29(1):165–78.

69. Ostaszkiewicz J, Johnston L, Roe B. Habit retraining for the management of urinary incontinence in adults. Cochrane Database Syst Rev. 2004;(2):CD002801.
70. Ostaszkiewicz J, Johnston L, Roe B. Timed voiding for the management of urinary incontinence in adults. Cochrane Database Syst Rev. 2004;(1):CD002802.
71. Fink HA, Taylor BC, Tacklind JW, Rutks IR, Wilt TJ. Treatment interventions in nursing home residents with urinary incontinence: a systematic review of randomized trials. Mayo Clin Proc. 2008;83(12):1332–43.
72. Ouslander JG, Griffiths PC, McConnell E, Riolo L, Kutner M, Schnelle J. Functional incidental training: a randomized, controlled, crossover trial in Veterans Affairs nursing homes. J Am Geriatr Soc. 2005;53(7):1091–100.
73. Holroyd-Leduc JM, Straus SE. Management of urinary incontinence in women: scientific review. JAMA. 2004;291(8):986–95.
74. Hay-Smith EJ, Herderschee R, Dumoulin C, et al. Comparisons of approaches to pelvic floor muscle training for urinary incontinence in women. Cochrane Database Syst Rev. 2011;12:CD009508. doi:10.1002/14651858.CD009508.
75. Qaseem A, Dallas P, Forciea MA, et al. Nonsurgical management of urinary incontinence in women: a clinical practice guideline from the American College of Physicians. Ann Intern Med. 2014;161(6):429–40.
76. Nygaard IE, Kreder KJ, Lepic MM, Fountain KA, Rhomberg AT. Efficacy of pelvic floor muscle exercises in women with stress, urge, and mixed urinary incontinence. Obstet Gynecol. 1996;174(1):120–5.
77. Herderschee R, Hay-Smith EJ, Herbison GP, et al. Feedback or biofeedback to augment pelvic floor muscle training for urinary incontinence in women. Cochrane Database Syst Rev. 2011;7:CD009252. doi:10.1002/14651858.CD009252.
78. Herbison GP, Dean N. Weighted vaginal cones for urinary incontinence. Cochrane Database Syst Rev. 2013;7:CD002114. doi:10.1002/14651858.CD002114.pub2.
79. Dumoulin C, Hay-Smith EJ, Mac Habée-Séguin G. Pelvic floor muscle training versus no treatment, or inactive control treatments, for urinary incontinence in women. Cochrane Database Syst Rev. 2014;5:CD005654. doi:10.1002/14651858.CD005654.pub3.
80. Dumoulin C, Hay-Smith J, Habee-Seguin GM, Mercier J. Pelvic floor muscle training versus no treatment, or inactive control treatments, for urinary incontinence in women: a short version cochrane systematic review with meta-analysis. Neurourol Urodyn. 2015;34(4):300–8.
81. Anderson CA, Omar MI, Campbell SE, et al. Conservative management for postprostatectomy urinary incontinence. Cochrane Database Syst Rev. 2015;1:CD001843. doi:10.1002/14651858.CD001843.pub5.
82. Berghmans B, Hendriks E, Bernards A, et al. Electrical stimulation with non-implanted electrodes for urinary incontinence in men. Cochrane Database Syst Rev. 2013;6:CD001202. doi:10.1002/14651858.CD001202.pub5.
83. Ayeleke RO, Hay-Smith EJ, Omar MI. Pelvic floor muscle training added to another active treatment versus the same active treatment alone for urinary incontinence in women. Cochrane Database Syst Rev. 2015;11:CD010551. doi:10.1002/14651858.CD010551.pub3.
84. Hollingsworth JM, Wilt TJ. Lower urinary tract symptoms in men. BMJ. 2014;349:g4474.
85. Macdiarmid SA. Concomitant medications and possible side effects of antimuscarinic agents. Rev Urol. 2008;10(2):92–8.
86. Chughtai B, Levin R, De E. Choice of antimuscarinic agents for overactive bladder in the older patient: focus on darifenacin. Clin Interv Aging. 2008;3(3):503–9.
87. Hesch K. Agents for treatment of overactive bladder: a therapeutic class review. Proc (Baylor Univ Med Cent). 2007;20(3):307–14.
88. Samuelsson E, Odeberg J, Stenzelius K, et al. Effect of pharmacological treatment for urinary incontinence in the elderly and frail elderly: a systematic review. Geriatr Gerontol Int. 2015;15(5):521–34.
89. Shamliyan T, Wyman J, Kane RL. Nonsurgical treatments for urinary incontinence in adult women: diagnosis and comparative effectiveness. Rockville: Agency for Healthcare Research and Quality (US); 2012. Report No.: 11(12)-EHC074-EF.

90. Martin-Merino E, Garcia-Rodriguez LA, Masso-Gonzalez EL, Roehrborn CG. Do oral antimuscarinic drugs carry an increased risk of acute urinary retention? J Urol. 2009;182(4):1442–8.

91. Fullhase C, Chapple C, Cornu JN, et al. Systematic review of combination drug therapy for non-neurogenic male lower urinary tract symptoms. Eur Urol. 2013;64(2):228–43.

92. Pagoria D, O'Connor RC, Guralnick ML. Antimuscarinic drugs: review of the cognitive impact when used to treat overactive bladder in elderly patients. Curr Urol Rep. 2011;12(5):351–7.

93. Gray SL, Anderson ML, Dublin S, et al. Cumulative use of strong anticholinergics and incident dementia: a prospective cohort study. JAMA Intern Med. 2015;175(3):401–7.

94. Myrbetriq- Food and Drug Administration. 2012 highlights of prescribing information. http://www.accessdata.fda.gov/drugsatfda_docs/label/2012/202611s000lbl.pdf. Accessed 26 April 2015.

95. van Kerrebroeck P, Chapple C, Drogendijk T, et al. Combination therapy with solifenacin and tamsulosin oral controlled absorption system in a single tablet for lower urinary tract symptoms in men: efficacy and safety results from the randomised controlled NEPTUNE trial. Eur Urol. 2013;64(6):1003–12.

96. Miller JM, Ashton-Miller JA, DeLancey JO. A pelvic muscle precontraction can reduce cough-related urine loss in selected women with mild SUI. J Am Geriatr Soc. 1998;46(7):870–4.

97. Friedman B. Conservative treatment for female stress urinary incontinence: simple, reasonable and safe. Can Urol Assoc J. 2012;6(1):61–3.

98. Rogers RG. Clinical practice. Urinary stress incontinence in women. N Engl J Med. 2008;358(10):1029–36.

99. Lipp A, Shaw C, Glavind K. Mechanical devices for urinary incontinence in women. Cochrane Database Syst Rev. 2014;(12):CD001756.

100. Suckling J, Lethaby A, Kennedy R. Local oestrogen for vaginal atrophy in postmenopausal women. Cochrane Database Syst Rev. 2006;(4):CD001500.

101. Lee YK, Chung HH, Kim JW, Park NH, Song YS, Kang SB. Vaginal pH-balanced gel for the control of atrophic vaginitis among breast cancer survivors: a randomized controlled trial. Obstet Gynecol. 2011;117(4):922–7.

102. Abrams P, Andersson KE, Birder L, et al. Fourth International Consultation on Incontinence Recommendations of the International Scientific Committee: evaluation and treatment of urinary incontinence, pelvic organ prolapse, and fecal incontinence. Neurourol Urodyn. 2010;29(1):213–40.

103. Wood LN, Anger JT. Urinary incontinence in women. BMJ. 2014;349:g4531.

104. Amundsen CL, Webster GD. Sacral neuromodulation in an older, urge-incontinent population. Am J Obstet Gynecol. 2002;187(6):1462–5. discussion 1465.

105. Cornu JN, Peyrat L, Haab F. Update in management of male urinary incontinence: injectables, balloons, minimally invasive approaches. Curr Opin Urol. 2013;23(6):536–9.

106. Garely AD, Noor N. Diagnosis and surgical treatment of stress urinary incontinence. Obstet Gynecol. 2014;124(5):1011–27.

107. Herschorn S, Steele DJ, Radomski SB. Followup of intraurethral collagen for female stress urinary incontinence. J Urol. 1996;156(4):1305–9.

108. Kirchin V, Page T, Keegan PE, Atiemo K, et al. Urethral injection therapy for urinary incontinence in women. Cochrane Database Syst Rev. 2012;2:CD003881. doi:10.1002/14651858. CD003881.pub3.

109. Lapitan MC, Cody JD. Open retropubic colposuspension for urinary incontinence in women. Cochrane Database Syst Rev. 2012;(6):CD002912.

110. The James Buchanan Brady Urological Institute, The Johns Hopkins University, The Johns Hopkins Hospital, and Johns Hopkins Health System therapy for stress incontinence. http://urology.jhu.edu/incontinence/stress_incontinence.php. Accessed 21 May 2015.

111. James MH, McCammon KA. Artificial urinary sphincter for post-prostatectomy incontinence: a review. Int J Urol. 2014;21(6):536–43.

To Fall Is Human: Falls, Gait, and Balance in Older Adults

Patricia Harris and Maristela Baruiz Garcia

To fall is human. When we are young, we scrape our knees, sometimes break a bone, and rarely injure our heads. As we age, however, the potential harms that a fall can produce (or signal) can be devastating. Older individuals are at greater risk for harm due to the age-related physiologic changes (increased sway, decreased joint mobility), higher rates of comorbid conditions, and decreased ability to recover. These factors can lead to marked functional decline, deconditioning, and increased risk of repeated falls.

Recent statistics show an increase in deaths in the USA due to falls among the elderly. According to the National Center for Health Statistics, from 2000 through 2013, the age-adjusted fall injury death rate among adults aged 65 and over nearly doubled from 29.6 per 100,000 to 56.7 per 100,000. (Although much of the increase can be explained by improved reporting, these rates nonetheless reinforce the impact of a fall-related injury on the elderly population.) In 2013, unintentional injury was the eighth leading cause of death among the elderly, with about ½ of those deaths occurring after a fall [1]. Additionally, the risk of death from a fall increases with age, from 14.1/100,000 in those aged 65–74 to 226.1/100,000 in those 85 years of age or older. The medical costs related to falls in the USA in 2013, according to the Centers for Disease Control, were $34 billion [2]. Falls are also a predictor of subsequent placement in a skilled nursing facility.

P. Harris • M.B. Garcia (✉)
Division of Geriatrics, Department of Medicine, David Geffen School of Medicine at UCLA, 10945 Le Conte Ave, Suite 2339, Peter V. Ueberroth Bldg, Los Angeles, CA 90095, USA
e-mail: magarcia@mednet.ucla.edu

© Springer International Publishing Switzerland 2016
L.A. Lindquist (ed.), *New Directions in Geriatric Medicine*,
DOI 10.1007/978-3-319-28137-7_5

One third of individuals over age 65 fall each year. An estimated 10–30 % of falls result in severe injuries, from deep lacerations and bruises to fractures (hip, pelvis, leg, ankle, wrist, shoulder, rib) and traumatic brain injury. The consequences are ominous. For example, in the year following a hip fracture, mortality rates increase approximately fivefold for women and eightfold for men, with an overall mortality rate of about 12 % [3]. Similarly, traumatic brain injury accounted for approximately 620,000 hospital admissions between 2000 and 2010, with over 11 % of these resulting in death [4].

Death is not the only fall-related outcome; a fall in the elderly is associated with significant decline in overall health and well-being, debilitating fear of another fall, and is associated with higher rates of nursing home placement. Of those who sustain a hip fracture, only 50 % return to their previous level of function within the first year, and 18 % are unable to walk [5]. A Dutch study found that both major and minor injuries were associated with decreased function and quality of life, including decreases in domains such as mobility, self-care, usual activities, pain/discomfort, and anxiety/depression [6].

The location of falls, and their etiologies, also differ among this age group. Individuals who report independence with activities of daily living tend to fall outside, tripping over hazards or irregularities in pavement. Those with restricted abilities to perform ADLs tend to have "frailty" falls inside, due both to intrinsic (balance, strength) and extrinsic (pet cat, throw rug) factors [7].

Fear of falling can be nearly as restricting as an actual fall, leading to decreased mobility and in limited social interactions [8, 9]. Fear of falling is also associated with depression and inability to perform ADLs [10].

Given the specialized nature of falls in hospitals and nursing homes, we will limit our focus on those falls that occur in community-dwelling elders.

Risk Factors for Falls

As we stated previously, a fall (and its sequelae) is a geriatric syndrome. Therefore, although we discuss some of the major risk factors for falls independently, they are in fact interdependent, and when evaluating the patient, we need to keep in mind the multiple factors that can lead someone to be at higher risk for falling. We also should be able to identify and target those at higher risk for an adverse outcome should there be a fall [11].

Age

Advancing age is a risk factor for falls. Not all studies have shown that it is an independent risk factor, but aging is a marker for other comorbid illnesses. In one survey, 13.4 % of 65–69-year-olds reported a fall in the preceding 3 months, whereas 20.8 % of those over 80 reported falling in the same time period. The risk of injury, such as hip fracture or traumatic brain injury, also rises with advanced age [12, 13].

Prior Falls

A previous fall is a major predictor of a subsequent fall. One report examined 11 studies in which multivariate analysis showed association between prior falls and future falls. In some cases, a history of one or more in a previous year was associated with two or more falls in the next year [13, 14].

Activities of Daily Living (ADLs) and Instrumental Activities of Daily Living (IADLs)

Individuals who have difficulty with basic ADLs (bathing, dressing, grooming, eating, ambulation, toileting) and IADLs (using the telephone, shopping, housework, food preparation, medication management, managing finances) (ADLs and IADLs) have an increased risk for falls [15]. Likely, deficits in these areas are markers for frailty and comorbid illnesses. A screen for impairments in ADLs can determine who is at higher risk for falls and injury.

Gait and Balance

Aging is associated with decreased postural control and increased sway. There is also age-related reduction in proprioception. Additionally, factors that would affect gait and balance such as lower extremity weakness, orthostatic hypotension, concomitant illnesses that result in decreased ambulation or proprioception (Parkinson's disease, stroke, chronic dizziness, osteoarthritis, diabetes, etc.) are associated with a higher risk of falls. Simple tests of gait and balance (unsteadiness with turning, sitting down, being pushed, or standing on one leg) or of gait (amount of sway, velocity of gait, deviation from a straight line) can determine if an individual has gait and balance abnormalities [16].

Cognitive Impairment

Cognitive impairment affects more than memory—it also affects many complex motor skills, including the ability to ambulate. Individuals with cognitive decline are at higher risk for falls and hip fractures than those who do not have cognitive decline [17, 18].

Medication Use

The studies that link fall risk to medication use are generally case–control prospective observational trials. Investigators also use data taken from large surveys and data sets such as the Behavioral Risk Factor Surveillance System (BRFSS) [19].

Some studies examine insurance (usually Medicare) reporting, linking an adverse event (e.g., hip fracture) to prescription data. The ethics of a randomized controlled trial, either by administering a medication of concern or by withholding a needed medication, precludes randomization in most settings. However, observational data, especially when viewed in the aggregate through meta-analyses or systematic reviews, are valid and provide much needed information [20].

Although it seems obvious that medications that can affect the central nervous system can also have an effect on an individual's risk for falls, it has been difficult to determine which medications have an impact on falls and which do not. Several recently published studies have been helpful in clarifying some areas of this complex topic; other areas require more work before clear recommendations can be considered.

Polypharmacy The use of even one medication has been associated with an approximate 30 % increased risk of falls compared to individuals who use no medications, and the risk increases with increased use of different medications such that those who regularly use four or more medications have a 120 % increased fall risk compared to those who use no medications. Of course, the reasons for these falls are not only due to the medications being used (in fact, some studies show that the type of medication used does not matter), but to the comorbid conditions that lead to multiple medication use. In the end, polypharmacy can serve as a marker for increased fall risk and can serve to alert the clinical provider caring for these individuals [21, 22].

Central Nervous System Drugs The use of these medications is very highly correlated with increased risk for falling. They include neuroleptics, antipsychotics, benzodiazepines (and near benzodiazepines such as zolpidem), and antidepressants. This class of medications is linked to a 50–70 % increased risk of falls [21, 23]. All patients who take these medications require careful observation and referrals as appropriate (e.g., physical therapy for strengthening, community exercise programs for gait and balance training).

Antihypertensives Reports that address the association between falls and antihypertensive medications have conflicting conclusions. A large 3-year prospective study of 4961 hypertensive individuals showed an increased risk of fall with injury among those who were receiving moderately intensive antihypertensive therapy (usually more than one agent), and the risk was greatest among those who had experienced a previous fall [24]. This finding was recently supported in a review of Medicare data, showing that initiation of a new antihypertensive was associated with a 36 % increase in serious fall risk [25]. In contrast, a 2015 prospective study of 598 individuals between the ages of 70 and 97 showed no increased risk for falls and antihypertensive use over a 1-year time period. Curiously, the report appears to assume the static use of medications as reported at the beginning of the study and does not address discontinuation or additions of medications [26].

Other studies show an increased risk of falls and fractures within the initiation period of medication use [27–29], suggesting that increased patient education may lead to increased caution during the first few weeks of medication use and thus reducing the incidence of falls.

With regard to whether certain classes of medications are either protective for falls (some studies have shown a protective effect for angiotensin receptor blockers and calcium channel blockers) or increase the risk for falls (diuretics), the data continue to be conflicting. Recent work did not find a correlation between any class of medication and fall risk (e.g., the risk was equal across all classes) [21, 24].

In short, recent studies suggest that two populations are at increased risk for falls if they take antihypertensives: (1) those who recently started a new medication and (2) those with a previous history of falls.

Opioids   Most studies link the use of opioid medications to anywhere between a 40 and 300 % increased risk of falls [30, 31], although the 2009 meta-analysis mentioned above did not find an association [21]. This class of medications requires close monitoring whenever prescribed. On occasion, the side effect of the medication and its relationship to a fall can be deceptive; for example, a person can take an opioid and develop constipation, which in turn causes bladder outlet obstruction and which then leads to delirium, a urinary tract infection, and sepsis, and then the fall occurs.

Nonsteroidal Anti-inflammatory Drugs (NSAIDs)   Several analyses show a correlation between NSAID use and fall risk, with most articles citing a 20–200 % risk of falls [32]. NSAIDs have been linked to worsening heart failure, edema, and renal disease, and it is likely because of these comorbid conditions that NSAIDs become risk factors.

Anticholinergic Medications

Many medications have anticholinergic activities. Over-the-counter medications include sedating antihistamines and oral decongestants. Prescription medications include SSRIs (fluoxetine, paroxetine), incontinence medications (tolterodine, oxybutynin), tricyclic medications (amitriptyline, nortriptyline), and antipsychotics (olanzapine, quetiapine).

A recent prospective population-based study that analyzed self-report of anticholinergic medications (verified by pharmaceutical records) and falls revealed a similar finding, at least for men: a previous fall and anticholinergic medication use was associated with a 250 % increase in the risk of an injurious fall [33]. Other reports show risks between anticholinergic use and cognitive decline, but there is little data on falls [34].

Vitamin D: Protective? Hype?

The recent explosion of articles regarding vitamin D and its protective effects for everything from bone health to brain health to cancer protection has made it difficult to assess the vast body of literature and find consensus. A recent NIH conference report summarized specific recommendations for primary care: (1) there is widespread evidence that vitamin D and calcium supplementation promotes bone health,(2) that vitamin D supplementation can prevent falls in the frail elderly, and (3)that research linking vitamin D to benefits for other diseases is inconclusive. Furthermore, it warns against over-supplementation, stating that levels of serum 25-hydroxyvitamin D are the best indicator of vitamin D status and that levels are likely safest below 50–70 ng/mL, but that classic toxicity syndromes (significant hypercalcemia, kidney and liver damage) are not seen until levels reach 200–400 ng/mL [35].

The American Geriatrics Society has recommended a 1000 unit/day supplement of vitamin D, which they feel will lead to a recommended serum vitamin D level when tested (minimum 30 ng/mL). They chose this dose because studies that link vitamin D supplements to reduced fall risk show *no* benefit for supplementation at 600 units/day [36].

Vision and Corrective Lenses

Low vision, of course, is a risk factor for falls. However, the means by which to correct vision may also affect falls. Unfortunately, many bifocals today have a built-in problem—visual distortion at the boundaries where the lenses meet. A 2010 randomized controlled trial showed that bifocals were associated with 40 % more falls than single vision lenses [37]. An observational study compared bifocal, trifocal, or progressive lenses with wearers of unifocal or no lenses. They found deficits among the multifocal lens wearers in tests of postural control and in the rate of falls, with an overall 30 % increased risk of one or more falls within a 1-year time frame [38].

Footwear

The few studies that compare bare feet, thick-soled shoes, and thin-soled shoes and the risk for falling conflict each other. One study found that 51.9 % of surveyed individuals reported that they were either barefoot, wearing socks, or wearing slippers when they fell, translating to an odds ratio of 2.27 (95 % CI 1.21–4.24) [39]. The study did not distinguish between barefootedness and wearing socks or slippers. Another study found that athletic and canvas shoes were associated with the lowest risk of falls. Athletic shoes generally have more components that are thought to improve gait and balance [40]. Most studies are of marginal quality and a good analysis of footwear is warranted.

Approach to Screening and Evaluation of Falls

Falls in older adults are generally a result of a combination of factors; the more risk factors present in an individual patient, the higher the risk of falling [41]. A thoughtful approach to the problem of falling in the elderly population requires understanding of the physiologic changes associated with the aging process; awareness of the various factors associated with an increased risk of falling; recognition of the functional, emotional, and economic consequences of falls as discussed above; as well as an appreciation of the older adult's preferred health goals and his or her comprehension of the necessary elements to achieve those goals. Time-constrained patient–clinician encounters pose a significant challenge when performing a comprehensive evaluation, particularly of older adults with multiple medical problems [42, 43] including falls. This reality creates the need for an individualized strategy that is efficient, effective, and implementable in actual practice. The following sections will address current recommendations regarding fall screening and evaluation in the clinical setting.

Screening for Falls and Fall Risk

Falls in older adults may not come to the attention of the clinician for a number of reasons. Patients and clinicians alike may erroneously assume that falls are a normal part of aging and are therefore non-preventable. Screening to identify older individuals at risk of falling is a recognized quality measure by the CMS Physician Quality Reporting System (PQRS), Medicare Annual Wellness Visit, Meaningful Use Incentive Program, as well as Accountable Care Organization programs [41]. The American Geriatrics Society (AGS) and British Geriatrics Society (BGS) recommend that all community-dwelling adults 65 years and older should be asked at least annually about history of falls, frequency of falling, and difficulties in gait or balance [44]. The US Preventive Services Task Force (USPSTF) endorses a brief screening of individual risk of falling for all adults age 65 and older in the primary care setting. It recommends identifying at-risk older adults based on three factors: history of falls, mobility problems, and poor performance on the timed get-up-and-go test [45]. It does not endorse a comprehensive, multifactorial fall assessment to be performed universally for community-dwelling older adults without risk factors, because the likelihood of benefit is deemed to be generally small.

The Centers for Disease Control developed the STEADI (Stopping Elderly Accidents, Deaths, and Injuries) tool, an easy-to-use resource for assessing and addressing fall risk in clinical practice based on the clinical practice guidelines on fall prevention jointly put forth by the AGS and the British Geriatrics Society and input from health-care providers [46]. This tool involves the use of a patient questionnaire as well as brief initial screening questions to assist in risk stratification and to identify older adults who may benefit from further gait, strength, and balance evaluation, in-depth multifactorial risk assessment, and intervention [47]. The screening questions involve asking about history of falls in the past year, feeling unsteady, and worry about falling. An affirmative response to any of the key questions directs the provider to perform a gait and balance evaluation (see algorithm below).

Evaluation

A reported history of a fall within the past 6 months or a positive fall risk screen should prompt an evaluation for gait and balance impairment. The presence of gait and balance impairment, two or more falls, or one fall with associated injury should be followed by a multifactorial risk assessment and an individualized fall prevention program depending on the risks identified (see algorithm below) [46].

Gait and Balance Assessment

The most valuable component in the initial examination of an older adult with a history of a fall is an assessment of integrated musculoskeletal function and postural stability. There are a number of tools available to the clinician in the evaluation of gait and balance. The timed up-and-go (TUG) test is easily performed as part of a routine examination and is the most widely recommended [48]. In this test, the patient is observed rising from a standard armchair, walking 10 ft across the floor (with an assistive device if needed) at a normal pace, turning around, and walking back to the chair and sitting back down. An older adult who takes ≥12 s to complete this task is at high risk of falling. Additionally, careful observation of the patient during this test may uncover impaired balance, shuffling gait, loss of arm swing, unsafe turning, and the improper use of assistive device.

The four-stage balance test is a simple means to assess balance. With the clinician standing close and ready to support the patient should he or she lose balance, the patient performs four progressively more challenging stances, with eyes open and without using an assistive device. First, the patient stands with his or her feet side by side. Next, the patient is instructed to place the instep of one foot so it is touching the big toe of the other foot. Third, the patient is directed to place one foot in front of another, heel touching the toe. Lastly, the patient is asked to stand on one foot. The patient is to hold each stance for 10 s without moving his or her feet or requiring support, before moving to the next position. An older adult who is unable to hold the tandem stance for 10 s is at increased risk of falling [46].

The functional reach test is another quick way to evaluate balance. This test is performed with a yardstick attached horizontally to a wall at the height of the shoulder. The subject stands so that his or her shoulders are perpendicular to the yardstick. He or she makes a fist and extends the arm forward along the length of the yardstick on the wall, as far as possible without taking a step or losing balance. The total reach is measured along the yardstick; inability to reach ≥6 in. (15.25 cm) indicates a significantly increased risk of falls [49].

Other tests available to evaluate integrated musculoskeletal function are more time-consuming to perform during routine primary care encounters. The performance-oriented mobility assessment (POMA or Tinetti Assessment Tool) is a validated method to evaluate gait and balance. It requires meticulous attention to multiple items scored during the test, including the ability to sit and stand from an armless chair, step length, step height, step symmetry, path deviation, and several other components [50]. The Berg Balance Test, a useful tool in rehabilitation settings, is a 14-item scale which includes assessment of the tandem stance, semi-tandem stance, and the ability of a person to retrieve an object from the floor from a standing position. Balance scores predicted the occurrence of multiple falls among elderly residents and were strongly correlated with functional and motor performance [51]. The components of the Short Physical Performance Battery (SPPB) such as the tandem stance, gait speed, and tandem stance are also predictive of falls [52, 53].

Algorithm for Fall Risk Assessment & Interventions

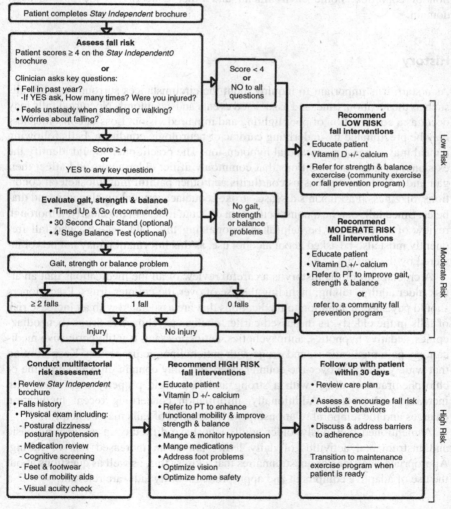

Centers for Disease Control (CDC) and Stopping Elderly Accidents, Deaths & Injuries (STEADI). (2015). *Algorithm for Fall Assessment & Interventions*. Retrieved July 22, 2015 from http://www.cdc.gov/steadi/pdf/algorithm_2015-04-a.pdf.

Multifactorial Assessment

A multifactorial risk assessment is recommended for all older adults who demonstrate an abnormality in gait and balance and a history of more than one fall or a single fall resulting in injury. A general knowledge of the risk factors associated with an increased risk of falling combined with what is known about the older adults' specific health conditions is helpful in developing an in-depth and individualized assessment and intervention. It is important to recognize that a good assessment encompasses elements beyond the biomedical realm which clinicians are typically more comfortable addressing in clinical practice. It may include evaluation of cognition, home environment, and other concerns in the psychosocial domain.

History

As a start, it is important to inquire about the circumstances surrounding the falls such as the location, time, and associated events and symptoms. Nocturnal falls may occur as a combination of poor lighting and impaired vision. Loss of consciousness may be precipitated by underlying cardiac or neurologic condition. Falls following a meal may suggest postprandial hypotension. The practitioner should identify the existence of medical conditions that commonly afflict older adults and affect their gait and/or balance such as osteoarthritis and other painful musculoskeletal conditions, dizziness, Parkinson's disease, stroke sequelae, cervical myelopathy, and diabetes. Since falls can be a nonspecific sign of acute illness in the elderly, a thorough review of systems can be helpful in recognizing this. Older adults who fall frequently must also be asked about alcohol use, as this information may not be volunteered by the patient.

A crucial part of the history is a careful review of all the medications that an at-risk older adult is taking, including the use of over-the-counter drugs. Practitioners should pay special attention to medications that are associated with an increase risk of falls in the elderly, as discussed earlier, such as psychoactive drugs (benzodiazepines, sedative hypnotics, antipsychotics, antidepressants), antihypertensive medications, pain medications, and drugs with anticholinergic properties. Keep in mind that widely available over-the-counter sleep aids may contain diphenhydramine or chlorpheniramine, drugs with a strong anticholinergic property associated with increased risk of fall. Additionally, information concerning recent medication changes and the temporal relationship with the onset of falls may be helpful.

Asmentioned previously, older adults who have difficulty in performing basic and instrumental activities of daily living are at an increased risk of falling. Appropriate questions or questionnaires that address this, as well as questions about the use of adaptive equipment and appropriate mobility aids, are relevant.

Physical Exam

In addition to the gait and balance assessment, an older adult with recurrent falls or a history of a fall with associated injury should undergo a more comprehensive physical examination. It should start with measurement of orthostatic vital signs to evaluate for postural hypotension. A focused examination of cardiac, musculoskeletal, and neurologic exam may uncover factors contributing to the falls and determine the appropriate intervention and fall reduction strategies. Foot examination is essential, and attention must be devoted to look for painful bunions and calluses, overgrown toenails, and poorly fitting footwear.

We also recommend cognitive screening. Cognitive impairment and dementia affect safety awareness and the ability to execute complex tasks. The Mini-Cog [54] can be used as a brief screen for cognitive impairment. Alternative cognitive screening instruments are the Montreal Cognitive Assessment (MOCA) [55] or the Mini-Mental State Examination (MMSE) [56]. However, they take longer to perform and may challenging to complete during a time-constrained office visit.

Consider visual screening through the use of the Snellen chart. If one suspects a hearing loss, a hearing screen can be performed by using a handheld audioscope or the whisper test. The association between impaired hearing and falls may be related to its effect on the older adult's ability to respond to auditory cues and attentional demands of the environment.

Diagnostic Work-Up

There are no studies that recommend routine laboratory testing after a fall or when a fall risk is evident. The decision to pursue diagnostic work-up must be guided by the clinical assessment. Holter monitoring, brain CT, echocardiogram, and other cardio-diagnostic or imaging procedures should be obtained only when indicated by the history and/or physical examination findings. When neither historical information nor physical examination findings suggest the cause of a recurrent fall, one may ask a patient to complete a detailed fall diary in order to identify patterns that uncover the etiology or contributing factors to the fall. Laboratory evaluation can rule out significant anemia, electrolyte abnormalities, hypothyroidism, and B12 deficiency when appropriate. Clinicians may be particularly challenged if the patient has cognitive impairment; she or he may not be able to provide an accurate history. In this instance, family members and caregivers can give useful collateral information.

Practitioners should also consider serum 25-hydroxyvitamin D levels as patients may benefit from vitamin D supplementation. A recent study, however, has put into question the relationship between vitamin D supplementation and reduced fall risk. At this time, however, since there is little risk in recommending vitamin D supplementation and monitoring vitamin D levels, continuing the current recommendations as mentioned above seems appropriate [57, 58].

Risk Factor Modification/Fall Interventions

Multiple strategies can be implemented to reduce the risk of falling. These interventions must be further individualized based on the modifiable risk factors identified during the in-depth assessment. The 2012 Cochrane systematic review, which included 159 randomized trials of interventions to reduce falls in community-dwelling older people and involved 79 individuals, reported that participants found a number of interventions that are likely to be beneficial in fall prevention [15]. Overall, exercise interventions, including multicomponent group exercises,significantly reduced the risk of sustaining a fall-related fracture among community-dwelling older adults. In addition, multifactorial interventions that included individual risk and home assessment, with home modification as appropriate, were effective in reducing the rate of falls. The review noted that home safety interventions appear to be more effective when provided by an occupational therapist.

With regard to procedural interventions, studies suggest that both initial eye cataract surgery and placement of pacemakers in patients with carotid sinus hypersensitivity reduce the risk of falling. Gradual withdrawal of psychotropic medication effectively decreased the rate of falls. Furthermore, a prescribing modification program for primary care physicians resulted in a significantly reduced risk of falls in their patients [59].

Of note, the Cochrane review concluded that overall, vitamin D supplementation did not reduce the risk of falls, but it may help reduce the risk in people with lower pretreatment vitamin D levels. Furthermore, it also found no evidence that cognitive behavioral interventions had an effect on the risk of falling. Fall prevention education alone, unaccompanied by interventions addressing other fall risk factors (e.g., exercise programs), is insufficient in significantly reducing the rate of falls.

Exercise and Risk for Falls

Many studies show that regular exercise reduces the risk of falls in the elderly. The American Geriatrics Society/British Geriatrics Society recommends that individuals at higher risk for falls be offered an exercise program that incorporates balance, gait, and strength training [44].

The Otago Exercise Program is a series of 17 strength and balance exercises delivered by a physical therapist in the home that reduces falls between 35 and 40 % for frail older adults. This evidence-based program, developed in New Zealand, serves as a model for successful community interventions to reduce the risk of falls [60, 61].

Recent studies on the effects of Tai Chi exercise on falls demonstrate significant reductions in fall risk in regular practitioners of Tai Chi. One randomized controlled trial found that a three times/week, 6-month Tai Chi program resulted in significantly decreased numbers of falls, particularly second falls and falls that led to serious injuries. Results of balance and gait testing improved over the course of the study, and these results persisted in 1-year follow-up [62]. Other studies support these findings [63].

In addition to an exercise program, other interventions to reduce the fall risk of the individual patient include the following:

Review Medications

In general, this is one of the most easily modifiable and effective risk factor interventions that a clinician can accomplish in the office setting. A general familiarity of the medications associated with increased risk of falling and knowledge of the at-risk patient's clinical conditions are essential in targeting the drugs that can appropriately be modified or discontinued. High-risk medications such as benzodiazepines, sedative hypnotics, antipsychotics, antidepressants, and antihypertensives should be carefully evaluated to determine if continued use is absolutely necessary.

Manage Postural Hypotension

Older adults with multimorbidity and polypharmacy may have multiple contributing reasons to have orthostatic hypotension, including disease states such as Parkinson's disease, diabetes, or dehydration; blood pressure-lowering medications such as antihypertensives and diuretics; and normal aging resulting in slow adjustment to position changes. Consider modifying the prescription program and having a good discussion with the patient with regard to risks and benefits of medications, lifestyle decisions, and living arrangements.

Address Gait and Balance Impairment

Gait and balance are affected by multiple factors: cerebellar function, vestibular function, proprioception, dementia, medication side effects, and so on. The clinician should always keep the factors that cause impairments in gait and balance at the forefront of clinical decision making.

Address Foot Problems and Footwear

Podiatry intervention, combined with foot and ankle exercises for older adults with painful foot problems, is helpful. Older adults at risk of falling should be advised to avoid shoes with higher heels and to use properly fitting shoes with high-contact surface area.

Address Vision Problems

For older adults with vision impairment, we recommend appropriate referral to vision professionals. However, it must be noted that interventions to treat vision problems have been shown to increase the risk of falls; the AGS/BGS cautions older adults with multifocal lenses to exercise more caution and to be more attentive when walking, especially on stairs.

One useful intervention, as we discussed earlier, is initial cataract surgery, which has been shown to decrease the risk of falling in older adults.

Modify the Home Environment

The primary care clinic is not equipped to evaluate and assist in home modifications, but referral for home safety evaluation (e.g., occupational therapists) when combined with multifactorial interventions may be appropriate for older adults with recurrent falls inside the home. Clinicians can suggest removal of loose rugs and other floor hazards (extension cords), installation of support structures such as grab bars and railings, as well as provision of adequate lighting.

Resources for Clinicians

A busy clinical practice cannot be expected to provide the full spectrum of interventions required to help their older patients reduce their risk of falls and fall-related injuries, nor is it easy to keep up with the vast amount of literature related to this topic. However, every clinician should feel comfortable with basic screening questions and examination tools and be able to guide his or her patient to helpful online and community resources (when they exist).

STEADI The Centers for Disease Control (CDC) has created a website devoted to what they have termed STEADI (Stopping Elderly Accidents, Deaths and Injuries) [46]. The website includes downloadable fact sheets, examination tips, etc., instructional videos for health-care practitioners (e.g., the timed get-up-and-go test), and materials designed for elders (and families) to download (e.g., the chair rise exercise). The site also includes links to other relevant resources.

National Council on Aging (NCOA)

The NCOA also provides tips on fall prevention and information on US federal interventions aimed at fall reduction, https://www.ncoa.org/healthy-aging/falls-prevention/. The 2015 National Falls Prevention Plan is actually a good summary of the state of the field, providing appropriate interventions to reduce the rate of falls in the USA [64].

American Occupation Therapy Association (AOTA)

The AOTA, https://www.aota.org/practice/productive-aging/falls/, provides a fall prevention toolkit, information on its fall project with the CDC, resources for Falls Prevention Awareness Day, and information on professional development resources, tip sheets, advocacy, and public awareness.

American Physical Therapy Association (APTA)

The APTA, http://www.apta.org/BalanceFalls/, provides information on balances, strength, and risks of falls. Information on specific conditions such as benign paroxysmal positional vertigo, balance and falls, and home safety tips are available.

American Geriatrics Society

The website, www.americangeriatrics.org, contains links to summaries of their recommendations for fall evaluation and prevention. Its sister website, www.HealthinAging.org, provides information to the public on numerous health concerns for the elderly, including fall prevention.

National Osteoporosis Foundation

The National Osteoporosis Foundation, www.nof.org, contains a wealth of information for both the public and the health-care practitioner regarding bone health, diagnosis of osteoporosis, treatment for osteoporosis, and advice on exercise for those who have osteoporosis.

Summary and Key Points

Patients may not see their fall history and fall risk as a medical problem. The healthcare provider can help patients modify their risks through screening, addressing modifiable risk factors, referring as appropriate, and being aware of community resources.

Changes in medications, eyewear, or footwear can lead to an increased risk of falls; caution individuals to be more aware when these kinds of changes are made.

Medications
– Review patient medications for polypharmacy (is there anything this patient doesn't need?), high-risk drugs, and over-the-counter medications.
– Warn patients of the increased risk of falls in the first month of starting new medications such as antihypertensives, psychoactive drugs, opioids, and anticholinergics.

Vision
- Multifocal lenses are associated with an increased risk of falls; most patients do not realize this.
- Cataract surgery, however, has been associated with a reduced risk of falls.

Postural Hypotension
- Patients can be educated to change position more slowly to avoid sudden blood pressure drops. This is especially true when patients get up from lying positions.
- Teach symptomatic patients to count to ten or sing a quick song prior to rising, after a position change.
- Reconsider (not) adding another antihypertensive in patients who already have a history of falls; the risk of injury is about equal to the benefit of better blood pressure control [24].

Vitamin D
- Vitamin D supplementation is inexpensive, relatively safe, and easily tolerated.
- The AGS recommends 1000 units daily; the USPTF recommends 800 units daily.
- There continues to be controversy regarding the efficacy of vitamin D supplementation, and recommendations may change.

Footwear
- Patients can be warned about slippery soles, stockinged feet, high heels, and the possible protective benefits of athletic-type shoes.

Exercise and Prevention Programs
- Studies show that it is difficult to implement an exercise or gait training program in the medical setting.
- Know your community and refer as appropriate.
- Tai Chi and Otago exercises have been shown to be particularly useful in fall prevention.
- Many communities have specific balance disorder centers that evaluate and treat gait disturbance.

Home Evaluation
- Physical and occupation therapists can generally evaluate the home through home health agency referrals.

Although the busy clinician may find it difficult to add yet another item on the to-do list of patient screening and prevention, a simple fall evaluation once a year, directed toward the at-risk population, can result in large patient benefits, with reduced loss of function, improved quality of life, and prolonged life span. It is certainly worth the time.

Key Points

1. One third of individuals over age 65 fall each year. An estimated 10–30 % of falls result in severe injuries, from deep lacerations and bruises to fractures (hip, pelvis, leg, ankle, wrist, shoulder, rib) and traumatic brain injury.
2. Individuals who report ADL independence tend to fall outside, tripping over hazards or irregularities in pavement. Those with restricted abilities to perform ADLs tend to have "frailty" falls inside, due to both intrinsic (balance, strength) and extrinsic (pet cat, throw rug) factors.
3. Risk factors for falls include advanced age, prior falls, difficulty with ADLs, gait balance irregularities, cognitive impairment, and medications.
4. Antihypertensive medications play a role in falls in older adults, with initiation of a new antihypertensive being associated with a 36 % increase in serious fall risk.
5. Eyewear can contribute to falls. Wearing bifocal or multifocal eyewear lenses is associated with 40 % more falls than single vision lenses.
6. Screening for falls and evaluation of gait and balance should be conducted annually for older adult patients with minimization of fall risk factors targeted.
7. Resources are available to improve gait and balance as a means of reducing falls.

References

1. Kramarow E, Chen LH, Hedegaard H, Warner M. NCHS Data Brief 199. Centers for Disease Control and Prevention. 2015. http://www.cdc.gov/nchs/data/databriefs/db199.htm.
2. Centers for Disease Control. 2015a. http://www.cdc.gov/homeandrecreationalsafety/falls/adultfalls.html.
3. Haentjens P, Magaziner J, Colón-Emeric CS, Vanderschueren D, Milisen K, Velkeniers B, et al. Meta-analysis: excess mortality after hip fracture among older women and men. Ann Intern Med. 2010;152:380–90.
4. Haring RS, Narang K, Canner JK, Asemota AO, George BP, Selvarajah S, et al. Traumatic brain injury in the elderly: morbidity and mortality trends and risk factors. J Surg Res. 2015;195:1–9.
5. Vochteloo AJH, Moerman S, Tuinebreijer WE, Maier AB, de Vries MR, Bloem RM, et al. More than half of hip fracture patients do not regain mobility in the first postoperative year. Geriatr Gerontol Int. 2013;13:334–41.
6. Hartholt KA, van Beeck EF, Polinder S, van der Velde N, van Lieshout EM, Panneman MJ, et al. Societal consequences of falls in the older population: injuries, healthcare costs, and long-term reduced quality of life. J Trauma. 2011;71:748–53.
7. Kelsey JL, Berry SD, Procter-Gray E, Quach L, Nguyen US, Li W, et al. Indoor and outdoor falls in older adults are different: the maintenance of balance, independent living, intellect, and Zest in the Elderly of Boston Study. J Am Geriatr Soc. 2010;58:2135–41.
8. Tinetti M. Fear of falling and fall-related efficacy in relationship to functioning among community-living elders. J Gerontol. 1994;49(3):M140–7. PMID: 8169336.
9. Austin N, Devine A, Dick I, Prince R, Bruce D. Fear of falling in older women: a longitudinal study of incidence, persistence, and predictors. J Am Geriatr Soc. 2007;55:1598.
10. van der Meulen E, Rixt Zijlstra GA, Ambergen T, Kempen GI. Effect of fall-related concerns on physical, mental, and social function in community-dwelling older persons: a prospective cohort study. J Am Geriatr Soc. 2014;62:2333–8.

11. Tinetti ME, Kumar C. The patient who falls: "it's always a trade-off". JAMA. 2010;303(3):258–66.
12. Stevens JA, Mack KA, Paulozzin LJ, Ballesteros MF. Self-reported falls and fall-related injuries among persons aged greater than or equal to 65 years--United States, 2006. MMWR. 2008;57(09):225–9.   http://www.cdc.gov/mmwr/preview/mmwrhtml/mm5709a1.htm. Accessed 08 Aug 2015.
13. Ganz DA, Bao Y, Shekelle PG, Rubenstein LZ. Will my patient fall? JAMA. 2007;297(1):77–86.
14. Deandrea S, Lucenteforte E, Bravi F, Foschi R, La Vecchia C, Negri E. Risk factors for falls in community-dwelling older people: a systematic review and meta-analysis. Epidemiology. 2010;21(5):658–68.
15. Gillespie LD, Robertson MC, Gillespie WJ, Sherrington C, Gates S, Clemson LM, et al. Interventions for preventing falls in older people living in the community. Cochrane Database Syst Rev. 2012; Issue 9. Art. No.: CD007146. doi:10.1002/14651858.CD007146.pub3.
16. Tinetti ME, Speechley M, Ginter SF. Risk factors for falls among elderly persons living in the community. N Engl J Med. 1988;319:1701–7.
17. Muir SW, Gopaul K, Montero Odasso MM. The role of cognitive impairment in fall risk among older adults: a systematic review and meta-analysis. Age Ageing. 2012;41:299–308. PMID: 22374645.
18. Amboni M, Barone P, Hausdorff JM. Cognitive contributions to gait and falls: evidence and implications. Mov Disord. 2013;28:1520–33. PMID: 24132840.
19. Centers for Disease Control. 2015b. Behavioral risk factor surveillance system. http://www.cdc.gov/brfss/. Accessed 08 Aug 2015.
20. Anglemyer A, Horvath HT, Bero L. Healthcare outcomes assessed with observational study designs compared with those assessed in randomized trials. Cochrane Database Syst Rev. 2014. doi:10.1002/14651858.MR000034.pub2.
21. Woolcott JC, Richardson KJ, Wiens MO, Patel B, Marin J, Khan KM, et al. Meta-analysis of the impact of 9 medication classes on falls in elderly persons. Arch Intern Med. 2009;169:1952–60. PMID: 19933955.
22. Pan HH, Li CY, Chen TJ, Su TP, Wang KY. 2014. Association of polypharmacy with fall-related fractures in older Taiwanese people: age- and gender-specific analyses. BMJ Open. http://bmjopen.bmj.com/content/4/3/e004428. PMID: 24682575.
23. Fraser LA, Liu K, Naylor KL, Hwang YJ, Dixon SN, Shariff SZ, et al. Falls and fractures with atypical antipsychotic medication use: a population-based cohort study. JAMA Intern Med. 2015;175(3):450–2.
24. Tinetti ME, Han L, Lee DS, McAvay GJ, Peduzzi P, Gross CP, et al. Antihypertensive medications and serious fall injuries in a nationally representative sample of older adults. JAMA Intern Med. 2014;174:588–95.
25. Shimbo D, Bowling CB, Levitan E, et al. Risk of serious fall injuries after initiation of antihypertensive medications in older adults (abstract). J Am Soc Hypertens. 2015;e15. http://news.medlive.cn/uploadfile/20150520/14320916542471.pdf. Accessed 08 Aug 2015.
26. Lipsitz LA, Habtemariam D, Gagnon M, Iloputaife I, Sorond F, Tchalla AE, et al. Reexamining the effect of antihypertensive medications on falls in old age. Hypertension. 2015;66:183–9. PMID: 25941341.
27. Butt DA, Mamdani M, Austin PC, Tu K, Gomes T, Glazier RH. The risk of hip fracture after initiating antihypertensive drugs in the elderly. Arch Intern Med. 2012;172:1739–44.
28. Butt DA, Mamdani M, Austin PC, Tu K, Gomes T, Glazier RH. The risk of falls on the initiation of antihypertensive drugs in the elderly. Osteoporos Int. 2013;24:2649–57.
29. Choi HJ, Park C, Lee YK, Ha YC, Jang S, Shin CS. Risk of fractures in subjects with antihypertensive medications: a nationwide claim study. Int J Cardiol. 2015;184:62–7.
30. Rolita L, Spegman A, Tang X, Cronstein BN. Greater number of narcotic analgesic prescriptions for osteoarthritis is associated with falls and fractures in elderly adults. J Am Geriatr Soc. 2013;61:335–40. PMID: 23452054.

31. Takkouche B, Montes-Martínez A, Gill SS, Etminan M. Psychotropic medications and the risk of fracture: a meta-analysis. Drug Saf. 2007;30:171–84. PMID: 17253881.
32. Hegeman J, van den Bemt BJF, Duysens J, van Limbeek J. NSAIDs and the risk of accidental falls in the elderly. Drug Saf. 2009;32:489–98.
33. Richardson K, Bennett K, Maidment ID, Fox C, Smithard D, Kenny RA. Use of medications with anticholinergic activity and self-reported injurious falls in community-dwelling adults. J Am Geriatr Soc. 2015. doi:10.1111/jgs.13543 (epublished ahead of print).
34. Fox C, Smith T, Maidment I, Chan WY, Bua N, Myint PK, et al. Effect of medications with anti-cholinergic properties on cognitive function, delirium, physical function and mortality: a systematic review. Age Ageing. 2014;43:604–15.
35. Taylor CL, Thomas PR, Aloia JF, Millard PS, Rosen CJ. Am J Med. 2015. doi:10.1016/j.amjmed.2015.05.025. PMID: 26071820 (available online ahead of publishing).
36. American Geriatrics Society Workgroup on Vitamin D Supplementation for Older Adults. Recommendations abstracted from the American Geriatrics Society Consensus Statement on vitamin D for prevention of falls and their consequences. J Am Geriatr Soc. 2015;62:147–52. PMID: 24350602.
37. Haran MJ, Cameron ID, Ivers RQ, Simpson JM, Lee BB, Tanzer M, et al. Effect on falls of providing single lens distance vision glasses to multifocal glasses wearers: VISIBLE randomised controlled trial. BMJ. 2010;340:c2265.
38. Lord SR, Dayhew J, Howland A. Multifocal glasses impair edge-contrast sensitivity and depth perception and increase the risk of falls in older people. J Am Geriatr Soc. 2002;50:1760–6.
39. Kelsey JL, Procter-Gray E, Nguyen US, Li W, Kiel DP, Hannan MT. Footwear and falls in the home among older individuals in the MOBILIZE Boston Study. Footwear Sci. 2010;2:123–9.
40. Koepsell TD, Wolf ME, Buchner DM, Kukull WA, LaCroix AZ, Tencer AF, et al. Footwear style and risk of falls in older adults. J Am Geriatr Soc. 2004;52:1495–501. PMID: 15341551.
41. Reuben DB, Herr KA, Pacala JT, Pollock BG, Potter JF, Semla TP. Fall prevention. In: Geriatrics at your fingertips. New York: American Geriatrics Society; 2015. 118 pp.
42. Abbo ED, Zhang Q, Zelder M, Huang ES. The increasing number of clinical items addressed during the time of adult primary care visits. J Gen Intern Med. 2008;23:2058–65. PMID: 18830762.
43. Fried TR, Tinetti ME, Iannone L. Primary care clinicians' experiences with treatment decision making for older persons with multiple conditions. Arch Intern Med. 2011;171:75–80. PMID: 20837819.
44. Panel on Prevention of Falls in Older Persons, American Geriatrics Society, British Geriatrics Society. Summary of the Updated American Geriatrics Society/British Geriatrics Society clinical practice guideline for prevention of falls in older persons and recommendations. J Am Geriatr Soc. 2011;59:148–57. PMID: 21226685.
45. Moyer VA, U.S. Preventive Services Task Force. Prevention of falls in community-dwelling older adults: U.S. Preventive Services Task Force recommendation statement. Ann Intern Med. 2012;157:197–204. PMID: 22868837.
46. Centers for Disease Control. 2015c. STEADI-older adult fall prevention. www.cdc.gov/steadi/.
47. Stevens JA, Phelan EA. Development of STEADI: a fall prevention resource for health care providers. Health Promot Pract. 2013;14:706–14. PMID: 23159993.
48. Podsiadlo D, Richardson S. The timed "up & go": a test of basic functional mobility for frail elderly persons. J Am Geriatr Soc. 1991;39:142–48. PMID: 1991946.
49. Duncan PW, Weiner DK, Chandler J, Studenski S. Functional reach: a new clinical measure of balance. J Gerontol. 1990;45:M192–7. PMID: 2229941.
50. Tinetti ME. Performance-oriented assessment of mobility problems in elderly patients. J Am Geriatr Soc. 1986;34:119–26. PMID: 3944402.
51. Berg KO, Wood-Dauphinee SL, Williams JI, Maki B. Measuring balance in the elderly: validation of an instrument. Can J Public Health. 1992;83 Suppl 2:S7–11. PMID: 1468055.
52. Guralnik JM, Ferrucci L, Simonsick EM, Salive ME, Wallace RB. Lower-extremity function in persons over the age of 70 years as a predictor of subsequent disability. N Engl J Med. 1995;332:556–61. PMID: 7838189.

53. Guralnik JM, Ferrucci L, Pieper CF, Leveille SG, Markides KS, Ostir GV, et al. Lower extremity function and subsequent disability: consistency across studies, predictive models, and value of gait speed alone compared with the short physical performance battery. J Gerontol A Biol Sci Med Sci. 2000;55:M221–31. PMID: 10811152.
54. Borson S, Scanlan JM, Chen P, Ganguli M. The Mini-Cog as a screen for dementia: validation in a population-based sample. J Am Geriatr Soc. 2003;51:1451–4. PMID: 14511167.
55. Nasreddine ZS, Phillips NA, Bédirian V, Charbonneau S, Whitehead V, Collin I, et al. The Montreal Cognitive Assessment, MoCA: a brief screening tool for mild cognitive impairment. J Am Geriatr Soc. 2005;53:695–9. PMID: 15817019.
56. Tombaugh TN, McIntyre NJ. The mini-mental state examination: a comprehensive review. J Am Geriatr Soc. 1992;40:922–35. PMID: 1512391.
57. LeBlanc ES, Chou R. Vitamin D and falls—fitting new data with current guidelines. JAMA Intern Med. 2015;175:712–3. PMID: 25799014.
58. Uusi-Rasi K, Patil R, Karinkanta S, Kannus P, Tokola K, Lamberg-Allardt C, et al. Exercise and vitamin D in fall prevention among older women: a randomized clinical trial. JAMA Intern Med. 2015;175:703–11. PMID: 25799402.
59. Milos V, Bondesson Å, Magnusson M, Jakobsson U, Westerlund T, Midlöv P. Fall risk-increasing drugs and falls: a cross-sectional study among elderly patients in primary care. BMC Geriatr. 2014;14:40. doi:10.1186/1471-2318-14-40. PMID: 24674152.
60. Liu-Ambrose T, Eng JJ. Exercise training and recreational activities to promote executive functions in chronic stroke: a proof-of-concept study. J Stroke Cerebrovasc Dis. 2015;24:130–7. PMID: 25440324.
61. Liu-Ambrose T, Donaldson MG, Ahamed Y, Graf P, Cook WL, Close J, et al. Otago home-based strength and balance retraining improves executive functioning in older fallers: a randomized controlled trial. J Am Geriatr Soc. 2008;56:1821–30. PMID: 18795987.
62. Li F, Harmer P, Fisher KJ, McAuley E, Chaumeton N, Eckstrom E, et al. Tai Chi and fall reductions in older adults: a randomized controlled trial. J Gerontol A Biol Sci Med Sci. 2005;60:187–94. PMID: 15814861.
63. Zhuang J, Huang L, Wu Y, Zhang Y. The effectiveness of a combined exercise intervention on physical fitness factors related to falls in community-dwelling older adults. Clin Interv Aging. 2014;9:131–40. PMID: 24453483.
64. Cameron K, Schneider E, Childress D, Gilchrist C. National Council on Aging Falls Free National Action Plan. 2015. https://www.ncoa.org/resources/2015-falls-free-national-falls-prevention-action-plan.

Should Your Older Adult Patient Be Driving?

6

Quratulain Syed and Ned Wilson Holland Jr.

Introduction

America is a nation of highways. The automobile is an integral part of modern culture and a source of income, recreation, and freedom for many. Practically, the ability to drive a car allows older adults to socialize in the community, shop for essentials, and take care of themselves without being a burden on others. Many older adults may have been driving for 70 plus years. As a result, driving cessation can result in social isolation and depressive symptoms in a former driver and additional burden on the caregiver. Most older drivers are responsible drivers and are less likely than younger drivers to drive recklessly, at high speeds, or under the influence of alcohol [1]. Unfortunately, chronic medical conditions may limit the ability to drive safely, and the burden of chronic disease increases with age. The Centers for Disease Control and Prevention (CDC) reports that in 2010, motor vehicle injuries were the second leading cause of injury-related deaths among 65–85 year age group. The Fatality Analysis Reporting System data indicates that individuals aged 80 and older have a higher rate of fatality and injury in motor vehicle crashes per million miles driven than any other age group except for teenagers.

Many clinicians are not comfortable discussing driving safety with older patients. However, in reality determining an elderly person's ability to continue driving rests

Q. Syed (✉)
Division of General Medicine and Geriatrics, Department of Medicine, Grady Memorial Hospital, Emory University School of Medicine, 49 Jesse Hill Jr. Drive, Atlanta, GA 30303, USA
e-mail: qsyed@emory.edu

N.W. Holland Jr.
Division of General Medicine and Geriatrics, Department of Medicine, Emory University School of Medicine, Atlanta Veterans Affairs Medical Center, 1670 Clairmont Road, Decatur, GA 30033, USA
e-mail: Wilson.Holland@va.gov

© Springer International Publishing Switzerland 2016
L.A. Lindquist (ed.), *New Directions in Geriatric Medicine*,
DOI 10.1007/978-3-319-28137-7_6

on physicians' shoulders. Therefore, clinicians are more receptive to education to improve their skills in office evaluation of the elderly drivers [2]. In this article, we'll review some common conditions in older adults that can affect driving skills, evidence-based guidelines for driving in these conditions, and how to assess for driving safety in your patient.

Neurocognitive Disorders and Driving

Cognitive impairment due to Alzheimer's disease (AD) can affect memory, attention span, problem-solving skills, multitasking, orientation, judgment, and reaction speed, which can impair driving skills. Individuals with AD have been observed to make more safety and lane observance errors than controls and have higher rates of motor vehicle accidents (MVA) when the driver's approach to an intersection triggers an illegal incursion by another vehicle in simulated driving evaluations [3, 4]. Even in amnestic mild cognitive impairment, defined as very mild short-term memory deficits and slight impairment in problem-solving without functional decline, driving skills such as lane control may be impaired [5].

Frontotemporal dementia (FTD) has been associated with profound impairments in reasoning, task flexibility, planning, and execution. Persons with FTD are more likely to drive poorly, including speeding, running "stop" signs, and suffering more off-road crashes and collisions than controls [6].

Individuals with HIV-associated cognitive impairment experience impairment in executive function and visual attention and therefore are also at a higher rate of MVA compared to HIV-positive individuals without cognitive impairment [7, 8].

The diagnosis of dementia is insufficient to predict a person's ability to drive safely. Therefore, The American Academy of Neurology has proposed using the Clinical Dementia Rating (CDR) scale to identify individuals with dementia at increased risk of unsafe driving, as there is a strong (Level A) evidence relating dementia stage to driving risk [9, 10]. In mild dementia (CDR score of 1) when memory loss is accompanied by moderate difficulty in problem-solving and functional impairment in complex activities of daily living, as few as 41 % of drivers may drive safely. There is poor correlation between an individual's self-rating or caregiver's rating of driving abilities as "safe," and an on-road driving test (Level A evidence). However, a caregiver's rating of an individual's driving skills as marginal or unsafe is useful in identifying unsafe drivers (Level B evidence). Other "red flags" include recent traffic citations, motor vehicle accidents, self-reported situational avoidance, mini-mental state examination scores of 24 or less, or emergence of an aggressive or impulsive personality (Level C evidence) (Table 6.1) [9]. With amnestic mild cognitive impairment (CDR of 0.5), most drivers "pass" the driving evaluation, but the red flags described above may be used to guide driver evaluation referrals. Moderate to severe dementia (CDR score of 2 and 3) may result in severe impairment in memory, judgment, and ability to do complex activities of daily living. Therefore, these patents should be strongly encouraged to stop driving and use alternative means of transportation.

Table 6.1   Identifying at-risk driving patterns in individuals with cognitive impairment

Level of evidence	Characteristics useful in identifying unsafe drivers	Characteristics not useful in identifying unsafe drivers
A	Clinical Dementia Rating score	Patient's self-rating of driving ability as safe
B	Caregiver's rating of driving ability as marginal or unsafe	
C	History of traffic citations or crashes	Lack of situational avoidance
	Reduced driving mileage	
	Self-reported situational avoidance	
	MMSE scores <24	
	Aggressive or impulsive personality	

The trail-making test part B (aka Trails B) which can be administered in 3–5 min highly correlates with recent or future at-fault MVA [11, 12]. It can be employed by clinicians to screen for fitness to drive in busy office settings.

A detailed neuropsychological assessment may be useful for evaluation of memory, spatial cognition, and executive functioning if questions about the diagnosis of dementia. However, there is insufficient evidence to support referral for neuropsychological testing to assess driving risk in patients with dementia.

There is no evidence to support or refute benefit of interventional strategies as driver rehabilitation for drivers with dementia.

Parkinson's Disease and Driving

Drivers with Parkinson's disease (PD) have been noted to have problems with lateral position on the road at speed below 50 km/h, speed adaptations at speed above 50 km/h, turning left maneuvers, lane keeping, observing their blind spot, backing up, parking, and negotiating traffic light [13, 14]. They also have poorer vehicle control in low-contrast visibility conditions as fog and are at higher risk for crashes in these circumstances [15].

Level B evidence exists for the useful field of view, contrast sensitivity, trails B and B–A (B–A = time on trails A subtracted from time on trails B), functional reach, and Unified Parkinson's Disease Rating Scale "off" motor scores for probably predicting driving performance [16].

Clinicians can perform functional reach test and trails B in their office for initial assessment. Individual with mild motor disability from PD may be fit for driving. They should be referred for a baseline driving evaluation upon diagnosis and then yearly for reassessment. There should be a plan to recommend cessation of driving and using alternate mode of transportation as the disease progresses. For individuals with severe motor impairment and disease severity, cessation of driving should be recommended [17].

Cardiovascular Diseases and Driving

Sudden incapacitation of the driver is estimated to be responsible for up to 3 % of all motor vehicle accidents, and approximately 10 % of these episodes are noted to be of cardiac origin [18]. Up to 35 % of all syncopal episodes while driving are neurally mediated and include neurocardiogenic syncope, situational syncope, and carotid sinus hypersensitivity constitutes. Cardiac arrhythmias (including bradyarrhythmias, supraventricular tachyarrhythmias, ventricular tachyarrhythmias) followed by ortho-static intolerance are other common causes of syncope while driving [19, 20].

Approximately 17–40 % of patients with history of syncope may have recurrences within a year of follow-up. In patients who have had a syncopal episode while driving, the actuarial recurrence of syncope is 14 % at 1 year. Driving restriction should there-fore be recommended for patients with recurrent or severe syncopal episodes, until a cause is identified and symptoms are controlled. As the causes and rates of recurrence of syncope are similar in patients who have it while driving and in those who have it while not driving, driving-related recommendations also apply to both [21]. Table 6.2 lists common cardiac arrhythmias and driving recommendations for those conditions.

Table 6.2 Driving recommendations for individuals with cardiac arrhythmias

Cardiac arrhythmias	Treatment	Driving restrictions	
		Private drivers	Commercial drivers
Symptomatic bradycardia	Discontinue offending medicine	After successful treatment	
	Pacemaker implantation	After 1–4 weeks	When pacemaker functioning appropriately
Supraventricular tachyarrhythmias	Medical treatment	After successful treatment	
	Catheter ablation	After successful treatment	After establishing long-term success
Ventricular arrhythmias	Medical treatment	After successful treatment	
	Catheter ablation	After successful treatment	After establishing long-term success
	ICD implant: primary prevention	4 weeks	Permanent
	ICD implant: secondary prevention	3 months (EHRA)	Permanent
		6 months (AHA)	
	Replacement of ICD	1 week	Permanent
	Replacement of lead system	4 weeks	Permanent
	Refusal of ICD: primary prevention	No restriction	Permanent
	Refusal of ICD: secondary prevention	7 months	Permanent

Adapted from Sorajja et al., Consensus statement of the European Heart Rhythm Association (EHRA) and the American Heart Association (AHA) and the North American Society of Pacing and Electrophysiology [21, 46, 47]

For patients who have implantable cardioverter defibrillator (ICD), device discharges are frequent. For individuals with history of ventricular tachycardia/fibrillation, 5 years actuarial incidence of appropriate ICD shocks ranges between 55 and 70 %. Also up to 30 % of individuals experience a syncopal or near-syncopal episode during an appropriate ICD shock [22]. However, in a survey of participants of Antiarrhythmics Versus Implantable Defibrillators (AVID) trial, none of the motor vehicle accidents were preceded by the driver receiving shock from ICD [23].

Polypharmacy and Driving

Two-thirds of people aged 65 and older take five or more medications daily. Psychoactive drugs (including benzodiazepines and tricyclic antidepressants) can result in impaired tracking and coordination, increased reaction time, and increase risk of MVA requiring hospitalization in older drivers [24]. Additionally, antiepileptics, dopaminergic medicines, muscle relaxants, hypoglycemics, antihistamines, and centrally acting muscle relaxants can affect the level of alertness and cause MVA [25]. The "Roadwise Rx" is a free online tool developed by American Automobile Association Foundation for Traffic Safety [26]. It allows a clinician (or patient) to enter the names of medicines and check if a medication can affect driving. Clinicians should also review their patients' medications periodically to eliminate unnecessary medicines and trim down the medication lists. The Beers List, "START" (screening tool to alert doctors to right treatment), and "STOPP" (screening tool of older person's prescriptions) tools can be useful in identifying potentially inappropriate medications [27, 28].

Vision Impairment and Driving

For safe driving, a driver should have adequate central vision to be able to see road signs, roadside objects, traffic lights, roadway markings, pedestrians, and other vehicles on the road, while the car is moving, under varying light and weather conditions. The driver should also have adequate depth perception and peripheral vision to be able to judge distance and speed and monitor objects and movement in the vicinity to identify possible threats in the driving environment. Central vision can be affected by age-related macular degeneration and cataracts, whereas glaucoma and strokes can affect peripheral vision. Cataracts can affect night vision and cause glare and contrast sensitivity.

The licensing authorities in the USA currently rely on visual acuity for vision screening for licensing purposes, which doesn't assess peripheral vision, visual attention, depth perception, and contrast sensitivity. Therefore, state laws pertaining to vision tests have not been associated with a lower fatality rate among older drivers [29]. Clinicians should counsel patients on their driving risk based on the diagnosis and treatment potential. Drivers undergoing cataract surgeries have been noted to have improvement in visual acuity and self-reported improvement in daytime driving up to 5 years after the surgery, though it doesn't significantly affect night driving [30]. Therefore, surgical correction of cataracts should be recommended to allow drivers with cataracts to continue driving.

Hearing Impairment and Driving

Moderate self-reported hearing loss, especially in the right ear, has been associated with higher rates of motor vehicle accidents among drivers aged 50 and older [31]. Drivers with dual sensory impairment are at a greater risk of motor vehicle accidents than those with only hearing or vision impairment [32]. Additionally, moderate to severe hearing impairment in older drivers is associated with worse driving performance in the presence of visual and auditory distracters [33].

Older adults with self-reported hearing impairment should be counseled to undergo hearing evaluation, followed by counseling to limit distracters during driving and use hearing aids if there is moderate hearing impairment. For those with severe hearing impairment or additional vision impairment, limiting driving and using alternate mode of transportation should be discussed.

Orthopedic Surgeries and Driving

A driver's ability to navigate steering wheel or apply brakes can be affected by an injury or a recent surgery of upper or lower extremities. Postoperative pain can also cause distraction and affect safe operation of a motor vehicle. The use of casts, slings, splints, and knee and elbow immobilizers can also affect an individual's ability to use the affected extremity to navigate the motor vehicle. Typically, impairment in driving ability is measured by changes in the time needed to perform an emergency stop. Recommendations regarding optimal time to resume driving after various elective or emergency orthopedics surgeries have been summarized in Table 6.3.

Table 6.3 Driving recommendations for individuals undergoing orthopedic procedures

Orthopedics procedures	When to resume driving
Knee arthroscopy (excluding ACL)	4 weeks
Right ACL reconstruction	4–6 weeks
Left ACL reconstruction	2 weeks
Right total knee arthroplasty	10 days- 8 weeks
Right total hip arthroplasty	6–8 weeks
Right ankle fracture	9 weeks
Bunion surgery	6 weeks
Major lower extremity fracture	6 weeks after initial weight bearing
Discectomy for radiculopathy	After discharge from hospital
Lumbar spinal fusion	After discharge from hospital

Adapted from Marecek et al. [48] and Goodwin et al. [49]

Physical Impairment and Driving Safety

Generalized physical debility as manifested by increased risk of falls can be a predictor of impaired driving skills, as both of these tasks require attention and ability to multitask. Individuals at high risk of falls, measured by Physiological Profile Assessment, have been noted to have a significantly slower response time to critical events during simulated driving assessment (400 ms slower) compared with low falls-risk drivers [34].

Epilepsy and Driving

Drivers with history of seizures run the risk of sudden incapacitation during a seizure episode, which can lead to harm to self or others if the driver is behind the wheels. However, this risk is very low if seizure disorder is controlled. Most studies show that drivers with history of seizures are not at any higher risk of MVA compared to drivers with other chronic medical conditions [35]. Physicians should refer to their state regulations governing reporting of epilepsy and breakthrough seizures.

Sleep Disturbance and Driving Safety

Sleep disorders including primary insomnia, obstructive sleep apnea (OSA), and circadian rhythm sleep disorders can result in reduced alertness, increased sleepiness during driving, and increased risk of MVA [36, 37]. A driver exhibiting moderate to severe daytime sleepiness and a recent unintended MVA or a near-miss due to sleepiness, fatigue, or inattention is a high-risk driver. For noncommercial drivers, treatment of OSA should be encouraged to reduce risk of drowsy driving. Compliance with continuous positive airway pressure (CPAP) for at least 4 h a night for >70 % of nights is recommended [38]. Also driving restriction should be recommended till symptoms improve. There is no compelling evidence to restrict driving privileges in patients with sleep apnea if there has not been a motor vehicle crash or an equivalent event. The American Thoracic Society clinical practice guidelines recommend against the use of stimulant medicines to improve alertness during driving in individuals with OSA [39].

It is recommended that commercial drivers should undergo a screening of symptoms of OSA during in-service evaluation and further evaluation as needed. They should also undergo out-of-service evaluation if observed or confessed excessive somnolence or road traffic accidents due to increased somnolence [40].

The Copilot Phenomenon

The copilot phenomenon describes a caregiver or partner of the driver who sits beside the driver when he/she drives and gives directions. This is an extremely important red flag to look for in the at-risk elderly drivers.

Evaluation

There are three key functions for safe driving: vision, cognition, and motor/somato-sensory function. The American Medical Association recommends assessment of driving-related skills (ADReS) test battery (see Table 6.4) which can be performed by a clinician in office to assess many key areas of the important functions which have been validated with driving outcomes [41]. It is important to note that ADReS is an assessment of important functional domains but is not a predictor of motor vehicle accidents. Additionally, a study by Ott et al. suggests that some of the ADReS may be better than others in assessing driving-related skills. In particular, trail-making test part B, rapid pace walk, and range of motion testing in office correlate best with on-road tests [42].

If there are concerns about a patient's ability to drive safely, clinicians can refer the patient to a certified driver rehabilitation specialist (CDRS) for driving assessment. The driving assessment usually includes an assessment of the driver's knowledge of traffic signs and laws, a cognitive assessment, a simulation test, and finally an on-road driving evaluation if deemed appropriate. Information about CDRS in your area can be obtained on the website of Association for Driver Rehabilitation Specialists (ADED).

In general, Medicare and other private insurances do not reimburse for driving services. The cost of driving assessment and rehabilitation is generally out of pocket and can vary from $100 to $500+ based on services provided and coverage provided by Medicare or private insurances, which varies from state to state.

How to Broach the Topic of Driving Assessment and Cessation During Your Clinic Encounter

Many older adults become defensive when driving is discussed, due to the fear that they may be asked to stop driving and may therefore lose their independence. It is best to discuss this issue directly in a non-confrontational approach, emphasizing your concern about your patient's safety and efforts to ensure that your patient can drive safely for as long as possible. Having a family member or friend present during the conversation can be helpful. It also helps reassuring your patient that a physician or occupational therapist doesn't have the legal authority to take away drivers'

Table 6.4 Assessment of driving-related skills (ADReS) in office

Components of assessment of driving-related skills (ADReS)	
Visual fields	Motor strength
Visual acuity	Trail-making test part B
Rapid pace walk	Clock drawing test
Range of motion	

Adapted from and available at: http://www.nhtsa.gov/people/injury/olddrive/OlderDriversBook/pages/ADReSscore.html

licenses. However, physicians should inform their patients about their responsibility to report to the Department of Motor Vehicle (DMV) medical conditions that may impair safe operation of a motor vehicle.

For many patients, driving cessation may not be the immediate goal, and focusing on options for safer driving such as not driving at night time and limiting driving to familiar areas may be sufficient for a period of time with close follow-up. When the clinician feels that the elderly driver is approaching the time to "give up the keys," discussing the importance of driving being a privilege, the safety of the patient and the safety of others should be emphasized. The American Medical Association suggests giving these drivers a prescription saying "Do Not Drive, For Your Safety and the Safety of Others." Focusing on alternatives that may allow them to stay connected with outdoor activities and developing alternative action plans with the elderly drivers and their families may reduce anxiety and depression that can develop when the elderly relinquish their driving privileges.

Reporting an Unsafe Driver

If a clinician believes that a patient has medical conditions that may impair safe operation of a motor vehicle, and put life of the patient or others at risk, the clinician should report to the local DMV in accordance with the state's mandatory reporting laws and standards of medical practice. The clinician should maintain the patient's confidentiality by ensuring that only the minimally required information is reported.

Follow-Up After Driving Cessation

Driving cessation can result in decline in overall health and increased depression in a former elderly driver who may have been driving for years [43–45]. Therefore, it is extremely important to follow up after counseling your patients to stop driving, to ensure that there is an alternative transportation option in place to allow the elderly to socialize and take care of their health and daily needs.

Key Points
1. There are three key functions for safe driving: vision, cognition, and motor/somatosensory function.
2. The licensing authorities in the USA currently rely on visual acuity for vision screening for licensing purposes, which doesn't assess peripheral vision, visual attention, depth perception, and contrast sensitivity.
3. The diagnosis of dementia is insufficient to predict a person's ability to drive safely.
4. There is no evidence to support or refute benefit of interventional strategies as driver rehabilitation for drivers with dementia.

5. In evaluating medications, the "Roadwise Rx" is a free online tool developed by AAA Foundation for Traffic Safety that allows a clinician (or patient) to enter the names of medicines and check if a medication can affect driving.
6. Moderate self-reported hearing loss, especially in the right ear, has been associated with higher rates of motor vehicle accidents among drivers aged 50 and older.
7. The copilot phenomenon, which describes a person who sits beside the driver when he/she drives and gives directions, is an extremely important red flag to look for in the at-risk elderly drivers.
8. If a clinician believes that a patient may be unsafe to drive, he or she should report in accordance with the state's mandatory reporting laws.

Abbreviations

ADReS	Assessment of driving-related skills
ADED	Association of driver rehabilitation specialists
CDRS	Certified driver rehabilitation specialist
CDR	Clinical Dementia Rating scale
CPAP	Continuous positive airway pressure
DMV	Department of Motor Vehicle
FTD	Frontotemporal dementia
ICD	Implantable cardioverter defibrillator
MVA	Motor vehicle accident
OSA	Obstructive sleep apnea
PD	Parkinson's disease
START	Screening tool to alert doctors to right treatment
STOPP	Screening tool of older person's prescriptions

References

1. Williams AF. Teenage drivers: patterns of risk. J Safety Res. 2003;34(1):5–15.
2. Marshall S, Demmings EM, Woolnough A, Salim D, Man-Son-Hing M. Determining fitness to drive in older persons: a survey of medical and surgical specialists. Can Geriatr J. 2012;15(4):101–19.
3. Rizzo M, McGehee DV, Dawson JD, Anderson SN. Simulated car crashes at intersections in drivers with Alzheimer disease. Alzheimer Dis Assoc Disord. 2001;15(1):10–20.
4. Dawson JD, Anderson SW, Uc EY, Dastrup E, Rizzo M. Predictors of driving safety in early Alzheimer disease. Neurology. 2009;72(6):521–7.
5. Griffith HR, Okonkwo OC, Stewart CC, Stoeckel LE, Hollander JA, Elgin JM, et al. Lower hippocampal volume predicts decrements in lane control among drivers with amnestic mild cognitive impairment. J Geriatr Psychiatry Neurol. 2013;26(4):259–66.
6. de Simone V, Kaplan L, Patronas N, Wassermann EM, Grafman J. Driving abilities in frontotemporal dementia patients. Dement Geriatr Cogn Disord. 2007;23(1):1–7.

7. Marcotte TD, Lazzaretto D, Scott JC, Roberts E, Woods SP, Letendre S, et al. Visual attention deficits are associated with driving accidents in cognitively-impaired HIV-infected individuals. J Clin Exp Neuropsychol. 2006;28(1):13–28.
8. Marcotte TD, Wolfson T, Rosenthal TJ, Heaton RK, Gonzalez R, Ellis RJ, et al. A multimodal assessment of driving performance in HIV infection. Neurology. 2004;63(8):1417–22.
9. Iverson DJ, Gronseth GS, Reger MA, Classen S, Dubinsky RM, Rizzo M, et al. Practice parameter update: evaluation and management of driving risk in dementia: report of the Quality Standards Subcommittee of the American Academy of Neurology. Neurology. 2010;74(16):1316–24.
10. Morris JC. The Clinical Dementia Rating (CDR): current version and scoring rules. Neurology. 1993;43(11):2412–4.
11. Stutts JC, Stewart JR, Martell C. Cognitive test performance and crash risk in an older driver population. Accid Anal Prev. 1998;30(3):337–46.
12. Ball KK, Roenker DL, Wadley VG, Edwards JD, Roth DL, McGwin G, et al. Can high-risk older drivers be identified through performance-based measures in a department of motor vehicles setting? J Am Geriatr Soc. 2006;54(1):77–84.
13. Wood JM, Worringham C, Kerr G, Mallon K, Silburn P. Quantitative assessment of driving performance in Parkinson's disease. J Neurol Neurosurg Psychiatry. 2005;76(2):176–80.
14. Devos H, Vandenberghe W, Tant M, Akinwuntan AE, De Weerdt W, Nieuwboer A, et al. Driving and off-road impairments underlying failure on road testing in Parkinson's disease. Mov Disord. 2013;28(14):1949–56.
15. Uc EY, Rizzo M, Anderson SW, Dastrup E, Sparks JD, Dawson JD. Driving under low-contrast visibility conditions in Parkinson disease. Neurology. 2009;73(14):1103–10.
16. Crizzle AM, Classen S, Uc EY. Parkinson disease and driving: an evidence-based review. Neurology. 2012;79(20):2067–74.
17. Classen S. Consensus statements on driving in people with Parkinson's disease. Occup Ther Health Care. 2014;28(2):140–7.
18. Petch MC. Driving and heart disease. Eur Heart J. 1998;19(8):1165–77.
19. Sorajja D, Nesbitt GC, Hodge DO, Low PA, Hammill SC, Gersh BJ, et al. Syncope while driving clinical characteristics, causes, and prognosis. Circulation. 2009;120(11):928–34.
20. Blitzer ML, Saliba BC, Ghantous AE, Marieb MA, Schoenfeld MH. Causes of impaired consciousness while driving a motorized vehicle. Am J Cardiol. 2003;91(11):1373–4.
21. Sorajja D, Shen WK. Driving guidelines and restrictions in patients with a history of cardiac arrhythmias, syncope, or implantable devices. Curr Treat Options Cardiovasc Med. 2010;12(5):443–56.
22. Freedberg NA, Hill JN, Fogel RI, Prystowsky EN, Group C. Recurrence of symptomatic ventricular arrhythmias in patients with implantable cardioverter defibrillator after the first device therapy: implications for antiarrhythmic therapy and driving restrictions. CARE Group. J Am Coll Cardiol. 2001;37(7):1910–5.
23. Akiyama T, Powell JL, Mitchell LB, Ehlert FA, Baessler C. Antiarrhythmics versus implantable defibrillators I. Resumption of driving after life-threatening ventricular tachyarrhythmia. N Engl J Med. 2001;345(6):391–7.
24. Meuleners LB, Duke J, Lee AH, Palamara P, Hildebrand J, Ng JQ. Psychoactive medications and crash involvement requiring hospitalization for older drivers: a population-based study. J Am Geriatr Soc. 2011;59(9):1575–80.
25. Orriols L, Delorme B, Gadegbeku B, Tricotel A, Contrand B, Laumon B, et al. Prescription medicines and the risk of road traffic crashes: a French registry-based study. PLoS Med. 2010;7(11):e1000366.
26. Association AA. Roadwise RX. www.roadwiserx.com. Cited 28 April 2015.
27. American Geriatrics Society Beers Criteria Update Expert P. American Geriatrics Society updated Beers Criteria for potentially inappropriate medication use in older adults. J Am Geriatr Soc. 2012;60(4):616–31.

28. Gallagher P, Ryan C, Byrne S, Kennedy J, O'Mahony D. STOPP (Screening Tool of Older Person's Prescriptions) and START (Screening Tool to Alert doctors to Right Treatment). Consensus validation. Int J Clin Pharmacol Ther. 2008;46(2):72–83.
29. Grabowski DC, Campbell CM, Morrisey MA. Elderly licensure laws and motor vehicle fatalities. JAMA. 2004;291(23):2840–6.
30. Monestam E, Lundquist B, Wachtmeister L. Visual function and car driving: longitudinal results 5 years after cataract surgery in a population. Br J Ophthalmol. 2005;89(4):459–63.
31. Ivers RQ, Mitchell P, Cumming RG. Sensory impairment and driving: the Blue Mountains Eye Study. Am J Public Health. 1999;89(1):85–7.
32. Green KA, McGwin Jr G, Owsley C. Associations between visual, hearing, and dual sensory impairments and history of motor vehicle collision involvement of older drivers. J Am Geriatr Soc. 2013;61(2):252–7.
33. Hickson L, Wood J, Chaparro A, Lacherez P, Marszalek R. Hearing impairment affects older people's ability to drive in the presence of distracters. J Am Geriatr Soc. 2010;58(6): 1097–103.
34. Gaspar JG, Neider MB, Kramer AF. Falls risk and simulated driving performance in older adults. J Aging Res. 2013;2013:356948.
35. Waller JA. Chronic medical conditions and traffic safety: review of the California experience. N Engl J Med. 1965;273(26):1413–20.
36. Arita A, Sasanabe R, Hasegawa R, Nomura A, Hori R, Mano M, et al. Risk factors for auto-mobile accidents caused by falling asleep while driving in obstructive sleep apnea syndrome. Sleep Breath. 2015;19:1229–34.
37. Barger LK, Rajaratnam SM, Wang W, O'Brien CS, Sullivan JP, Qadri S, et al. Common sleep disorders increase risk of motor vehicle crashes and adverse health outcomes in firefighters. J Clin Sleep Med. 2015;11:233–40.
38. Ayas N, Skomro R, Blackman A, Curren K, Fitzpatrick M, Fleetham J, et al. Obstructive sleep apnea and driving: a Canadian Thoracic Society and Canadian Sleep Society position paper. Can Respir J. 2014;21(2):114–23.
39. Strohl KP, Brown DB, Collop N, George C, Grunstein R, Han F, et al. An official American Thoracic Society Clinical Practice Guideline: sleep apnea, sleepiness, and driving risk in noncommercial drivers. An update of a 1994 Statement. Am J Respir Crit Care Med. 2013;187(11):1259–66.
40. Hartenbaum N, Collop N, Rosen IM, Phillips B, George CF, Rowley JA, et al. Sleep apnea and commercial motor vehicle operators: statement from the joint task force of the American College of Chest Physicians, the American College of Occupational and Environmental Medicine, and the National Sleep Foundation. Chest. 2006;130(3):902–5.
41. Association AM. ADReS. http://www.nhtsa.gov/people/injury/olddrive/OlderDriversBook/pages/Contents.html. Cited 28 April 2015.
42. Ott BR, Davis JD, Papandonatos GD, Hewitt S, Festa EK, Heindel WC, et al. Assessment of driving-related skills prediction of unsafe driving in older adults in the office setting. J Am Geriatr Soc. 2013;61(7):1164–9.
43. Marottoli RA, Mendes de Leon CF, Glass TA, Williams CS, Cooney Jr LM, Berkman LF, et al. Driving cessation and increased depressive symptoms: prospective evidence from the New Haven EPESE. Established Populations for Epidemiologic Studies of the Elderly. J Am Geriatr Soc. 1997;45(2):202–6.
44. Ragland DR, Satariano WA, MacLeod KE. Driving cessation and increased depressive symptoms. J Gerontol A Biol Sci Med Sci. 2005;60(3):399–403.
45. Edwards JD, Lunsman M, Perkins M, Rebok GW, Roth DL. Driving cessation and health trajectories in older adults. J Gerontol A Biol Sci Med Sci. 2009;64(12):1290–5.
46. Task force members, Vijgen J, Botto G, Camm J, Hoijer CJ, Jung W, et al. Consensus statement of the European Heart Rhythm Association: updated recommendations for driving by patients with implantable cardioverter defibrillators. Europace. 2009;11(8):1097–107.

47. Epstein AE, Baessler CA, Curtis AB, Estes 3rd NA, Gersh BJ, Grubb B, et al. Addendum to "Personal and public safety issues related to arrhythmias that may affect consciousness: implications for regulation and physician recommendations: a medical/scientific statement from the American Heart Association and the North American Society of Pacing and Electrophysiology": public safety issues in patients with implantable defibrillators: a scientific statement from the American Heart Association and the Heart Rhythm Society. Circulation. 2007;115(9):1170–6.
48. Marecek GS, Schafer MF. Driving after orthopaedic surgery. J Am Acad Orthop Surg. 2013;21(11):696–706.
49. Goodwin D, Baecher N, Pitta M, Letzelter J, Marcel J, Argintar E. Driving after orthopedic surgery. Orthopedics. 2013;36(6):469–74.

Making House Calls: Treating Older Adults at Home

Linda V. DeCherrie, Melissa Dattalo, Ming Jang, and Rachel K. Miller

The Importance of House Calls

Prior to World War II, physician house calls were the primary mode of health-care delivery in the USA and Europe. Almost all the tools a physician used regularly could be easily transported to the bedside. In addition, physicians often had more access to transportation and could get to their patients [1]. In 1930, 30 % of physician encounters were in the home, by 1950 only 10 % and less than 1 % in 1980 [2, 3]. In Europe, house calls continue to have a stronger presence than in the USA. In England, for example, physicians currently make ten times the number of house calls compared to the USA and 100 times as many to patients over 85 years of age [4, 5].

After World War II, physician house calls seemingly fell out of favor [6]. Many factors influenced a change in health-care delivery. First, technological advancements—such as development of x-ray technology—often required patients to come

L.V. DeCherrie
Department of Geriatrics and Palliative Medicine, Mount Sinai Medical Center,
1 Gustave L Levy Place, Box 1216, New York, NY 10028, USA
e-mail: linda.decherrie@mountsinai.org

M. Dattalo
Geriatric Research Education and Clinical Center (GRECC), William S. Middleton Memorial
VA Hospital and University of Wisconsin-Madison School of Medicine and Public Health,
2500 Overlook Terrace, 11G, Madison, WI 53705, USA
e-mail: mdattalo@uwhealth.org

M. Jang • R.K. Miller (✉)
Division of Geriatrics, Perelman School of Medicine, Hospital of the University of
Pennsylvania, 3615 Chestnut Street, Philadelphia, PA 19104, USA
e-mail: ming.jang@uphs.upenn.edu; Rachel.Miller@uphs.upenn.edu

© Springer International Publishing Switzerland 2016
L.A. Lindquist (ed.), *New Directions in Geriatric Medicine*,
DOI 10.1007/978-3-319-28137-7_7

to the hospital or clinic to get diagnosed or treated. In addition, the rise in physician specialization coincided with changes in payment systems, both of which influenced the number of house calls delivered in the USA.

Physicians who currently provide house calls in the USA are usually primary care physicians [6]. They must generally pick up the necessary skills for this practice through "on-the-job training"; few doctors receive any training in house calls in medical school or residency. In the 1990s, only 66 of 123 medical schools exposed their students to more than 1 hour on home care, and even fewer received training on actual home visits [7].

This must change, and recent changes in physician reimbursements suggest that the government agrees. There are approximately 400,000–2,000,000 homebound persons in the USA and another 1.1 million who are semi-homebound [8]. In 1998, Medicare established new billing codes for house calls and increased reimbursement for house calls by 50 %. In 2001, the reimbursement to assisted living home visits similarly increased. The number of house calls continues to grow slowly, but house calls remain less than 1 % of outpatient billing [9].

Increasingly, the question arises: Why aren't house calls expanding faster? There are many advantages to house calls for the appropriate patient. Patients, families, providers, and reimbursement systems all can benefit from house calls. For some patients with frailty, severe mobility impairment, or terminal conditions, getting to the physician's office is extremely taxing. For patients with dementia or psychiatric disorders, leaving the home can cause behavioral disturbance or paranoia [6]. Finally, families and caregivers are often better integrated into the care plan because of the on-site communication with the provider.

Providers can also improve the quality of their care by making house calls. Being in the home can give great insight into the medical issues with the patient from falls, to weight loss, and missed diagnoses. Technological limitations are evaporating. Today, almost all that is done in a primary care office can be done at home. Providers can use laptops or tablets to access medical records, while pulse ox's, ultrasounds, X-rays, and labs can all be done in the home.

Financially, house calls make good economic sense in an era of spiraling healthcare costs. The homebound patients are often some of the costliest in the health-care system. By providing care in the home, this cost can often be reduced. Recently, the results of the first year of Independence at Home Medicare Demonstration saved Medicare over $25,000,000, with an average over $3000 per beneficiary in the first year [10].

Who Can Participate in House Calls?

Any practicing provider can perform a home visit, even if he/she is not specifically affiliated with a home-based primary care practice. Home visits can be performed once, as part of a comprehensive assessment, or longitudinally over time, as part of a home-based primary care practice.

It is a common misconception that a patient needs to meet Medicare's definition of being "homebound" in order to receive a clinical home visit. While chronically homebound individuals compose the majority of longitudinal home-based primary care patient panels, there are many circumstances in which patients who usually attend office visits can benefit from home visits. Home visits may be appropriate to assess the home environment, to assess caregiver function, to verify eligibility for home health services in a face-to-face encounter, to negotiate clinical decision-making during a family meeting, or simply to meet a patient or caregiver request [11].

If a patient meets Medicare's two criteria for "homebound status," he/she may be eligible to receive ongoing home visits or home-based primary care. Patients can fully meet the "homebound status" criteria even if they leave the house for medical care or if they leave the house for other reasons that are "infrequent" or "of short duration" such as attendance at religious services [12].

Providers can receive fee-for-service Medicare reimbursements for home visits as long as they document why the visit needs to be conducted in the home rather than in the office. Otherwise, documentation for new patients in the home (99341–99345) or domiciliary/assisted living home (99324–99328) and established patients in the home (99347–99350) or domiciliary/assisted living home (99334–99337) is similar to the documentation required for evaluation and management office visits [11]. Medicare reimbursements for home or domiciliary/assisted living home visits are slightly higher than office visits of similar complexity, but the volume of home visits that can be completed in a single day is limited. That differential likely accounts for the fact that the volume of home visits that can be completed in a single day is limited by travel time.

Preparing for a House Call

Almost all evaluation and diagnostic services typically available to patients in clinics can also be made available to them in the home. Providers should bring portable equipment to assess vital signs, including a manual blood pressure cuff, stethoscope, pulse oximeter, thermometer, and a watch that counts seconds. Practices with high volumes of house calls often have home visit kits containing hand sanitizer, gloves, wound care supplies, phlebotomy equipment, sharps containers, sterile specimen cups, glucometers, tongue depressors, otoscopes, cerumen spoons to remove ear wax, lubricant, and fecal occult blood cards [11]. Providers may bring additional vaccines or any additional equipment needed for procedures (i.e., joint aspiration/injection). There are even portable electrocardiogram, echocardiogram, and ultrasound supplies. Community-based companies can provide home radiology services including chest X-rays.

Basic House Call Supplies

The house call clinician will need at his or her disposal basic medical supplies:
1. Medical equipment
Stethoscope
Otoscope
Ophthalmoscope
Tongue depressors
Sphygmomanometer
Thermometer
Sterile gloves, hand sanitizer, droplet mask
2. Phlebotomy/procedure/micro equipment
Gauze, 11 and 10 scalpels, medical tape, Steri-Strips, iodine, wound packing strips, alcohol pads, Band-Aids, chuck pads
Butterfly IV catheter tubing, phlebotomy tube holder with appropriate adaptor, and phlebotomy tubes with patient labels
Rapid viral swab, viral culture media
Blood culture vials, urine dipsticks, and culture vials
18, 20, and 22 gauge needles
5, 10, 25 cc syringes
3. Medications
Lidocaine
Solu-Medrol (or any other liquid steroid solution)
Tylenol, aspirin, clonidine, specific antibiotics
Sterile saline solution
4. Documents
Procedural consent forms
Advanced directives paperwork
POLST/MOLST forms

Labs and Imaging Resources

In some areas, phlebotomy services or home nursing are able to come to the home to perform blood work. While not mandatory, some house call groups train providers in basic phlebotomy. This minimizes resource use by incorporating obtaining blood work into the home visit.

The clinician should be aware of local mobile imaging resources as well. Often, home visit groups contract with mobile imaging companies to provide these services, which include X-rays, ultrasounds, EKGs, and, in some areas, Holter monitors, echocardiograms, bone density scans, and sleep studies. Imaging like CT scans, MRIs, and PET scans at this point still need to be done in a radiology suite. The results of basic studies like EKGs and X-rays may be interpreted by the home care clinician, but a contracted radiology or cardiology group should be considered for more advanced imaging. For more frequent blood work like INR checks, it may be reasonable to utilize a visiting nurse agency or for the practice to invest in a point of care INR machine.

With the advent of smartphone, technology can ease the financial burden of relying on these mobile imaging companies. While these mobile resources are of indispensable value, it may take several hours, potentially even a day, to obtain the workup needed—this does not include the time needed for the data to be read by a specialist. Smartphone and wireless technology has become increasingly sophisticated over time. Such devices include smartphone ECGs, otoscope, ultrasound probe, and glucometers.

In addition to examination and laboratory equipment, providers should consider what supplies they need for reference, prescription, and documentation. Documentation can be done via portable dictation devices or, when Internet is available, via laptops or tablets. Even if providers are using portable laptops and electronic medical records, they should be prepared to function without wireless Internet access during the home visit. This may entail bringing paper prescription pads, patient handouts with community resources, reference cards with clinic phone numbers, clinical assessment tools (i.e., mini-mental status examination), and pharmacologic reference books or smartphones with clinical reference apps.

House Call Safety Considerations

Safety precautions must be considered while preparing to conduct a home visit. The occupational risks of home health workers include road hazards while driving, biological hazards, latex sensitivity, patient lifting, hostile animals, and unhygienic or dangerous conditions [13]. For full-time home health-care workers, the rate of non-fatal assaults by people or animals is double the national average, and the rate of injury from motor vehicle accidents is ten times as high as hospital workers [13]. Basic safety precautions can include keeping supplies and personal belongings locked in the trunk of your vehicle, waiting to enter a home until the owner has control of all pets, attending home visits in pairs, carrying a cell phone for emergency communication, keeping office staff informed of your whereabouts, and being prepared to leave any situation in which you feel uncomfortable.

In addition, home visits present unique safety risks to the patients themselves. Portable equipment should be available, such as hand sanitizer, to ensure adequate hygiene, personal protective equipment necessary for standard precautions, and rigid biohazard containers for disposal of needles and other sharp instruments. In addition, pests may be present in unsanitary conditions and may contaminate equipment. Providers need to be prepared to confront all of these situations.

Performing the House Call and Conducting Assessments in the Home

House calls offer opportunities for more comprehensive assessments that typically can be accomplished during an office visit. The American Medical Association Home Care Advisory Panel offers guidelines on specific assessments commonly conducted in the home setting: functional, sensory, cognitive, psychosocial, nutritional, medication use, caregiver, environmental, community, and financial assessments [14]. Conducting visits in the home setting may also facilitate discussions about advanced care planning or serve as a bridge to hospice for patients with advanced illness. In fact, home visits are associated with increased rates of hospice referral and reductions in emergency department visits and hospitalizations [6].

One of the hallmarks of house calls is the ability to assess a patient's functional status in the context of his/her usual environment. Rather than just *asking* about patients' abilities to perform basic activities of daily living (ADLs), house call providers can actually observe them. ADLs include ambulating, bathing (i.e., can observe a patient climbing in and out of a bathtub), toileting, dressing, feeding, transferring (i.e., transferring from a bed to a wheelchair), and bowel or bladder continence. House calls also offer a unique opportunity for medication reconciliation and medication use assessment. Patients or caregivers can demonstrate the systems they use for managing medications from the pill bottles to the point of administration. In addition to medication management, other important instrumental activities of daily living (iADLs) to assess include using the telephone, arranging transportation, doing housework, shopping, and handling finances [14].

Assessment of cognitive function and decision-making capacity is also a key component of house calls. Memory difficulties, dementia, and neuropsychiatric symptoms (i.e., depression, confusion, agitation) are common among house call patients [6]. Since the primary goal of many house call patients is to continue living independently in their homes, providers must continually assess (1) the risks and benefits of remaining at home, (2) whether adequate in-home supports are available, and (3) any signs of self-neglect [6]. Clinical tools such as the Aid to Capacity Evaluation can guide the evaluation of a patient's decision-making capacity [15].

House calls also provide a critical window into patients' environments and support networks. Providers who perform house calls are often better able to coordinate with informal caregivers and other home health services [6]. Signs of caregiver stress may be more apparent in the home, and personal care techniques can be demonstrated in a real-world environment. House calls offer the ability to observe patients interacting with their caregivers and their usual environments. For example, a home care provider may notice that a patient's house is so cluttered that her walker cannot fit in the hallway. Consequently, instead of using her walker at home, she may brace herself on furniture or stacked boxes lining the hall. Beyond environmental fall hazards, other home safety concerns may be identified during home visits including inadequate food supplies, lack of running water, extremes of temperature, and rodent or insect infestations. Caring for patients in their home environments can offer unique perspectives into their daily lives, physical environments, and social support networks.

Managing Home Care Referrals/Partnerships

The home care clinician is also adept at utilizing and managing available community resources. To start, becoming familiar with available resources is a key step:

1. Area Agency on Aging: Most counties in the USA have an associated Area Agency on Aging, which provides valuable home resources, ranging from home health aides and case management to meals on wheels programs, access to transportation to appointments, and home repair.
2. Visiting Nurses Association: There are also local visiting nurses associations as well which provide skilled care (e.g., wound care, infusions, blood pressure monitoring, home safety evaluations) to patients. They are also able to make referrals to therapy.
3. Physical therapy and occupational therapy: Certain physical therapy and occupational therapy groups also equipped to do home visits for evaluation and treatment. It is useful to keep in mind that occupational therapists are also able to do home safety evaluations.
4. Social service networks are also available and vary depending on the specific region.
   (a) ElderNet is a great example of this in the suburban Philadelphia area.
5. Adult Day Care and LIFE programs: These are excellent options which can provide daytime supervision for functionally dependent, chronically ill, and/or cognitively impaired adult. This can provide significant relief of caregiver burden for daytime care.
6. Visiting specialists: Depending on the area, certain visiting specialists also do home visits. This service may include dentistry, optometry, podiatry, and psychology.

Each program has its own eligibility requirements, and a waiting list, so it is reasonable to start the application process earlier to ensure timely processing.

As one's home care practice becomes embedded in the community, keeping a close relationship with key organizations for resources is a mutually beneficial alliance. This direct communication, which can be done via telephone and email, not only decreases fragmentation of care but allows for excellent communication between health-care providers who see the same patient in different encounters and can serve as accessory eyes and ears to the primary home care clinician who quarterbacks the homebound patient's overall care.

Key Points
1. Any practicing provider can perform a home visit, even if he/she is not specifically affiliated with a home-based primary care practice.
2. If a patient meets Medicare's two criteria for "homebound status," he/she may be eligible to receive ongoing home visits or home-based primary care. Patients can fully meet the "homebound status" criteria even if they leave the house for medical care or if they leave the house for other reasons that are "infrequent" or "of short duration" such as attendance at religious services.
3. Providers can receive fee-for-service Medicare reimbursements for home visits as long as they document why the visit needs to be conducted in the home rather than in the office.
4. Documentation for home visits is similar to the documentation required for office visits, but Medicare reimburses for home visits higher than office visits of similar complexity.
5. Almost all evaluation and diagnostic services typically available to patients in clinics can also be made available to them in the home.
6. House calls offer opportunities for more comprehensive assessments that typically can be accomplished during an office visit.
7. Home care clinicians should be adept at utilizing and managing available community resources to meet the needs of their patients.

References

1. DeCherrie LV, Soriano T, Hayashi J. Home-based primary care: a needed primary-care model for vulnerable populations. Mt Sinai J Med. 2012;79:425–32.
2. Star P. The social transformation of American medicine. New York: Basic Books; 1982. p. 359.
3. Driscoll CE. Is there a doctor in the house? Am Academy Home Care Physicians News. 1991;3:7–8.
4. Meyer GS, Gibbons RV. House calls to the elderly- a vanishing practice among physicians. N Engl J Med. 1997;337:1815–20.
5. Aylin P, Majeed FA, Cook DG, et al. Home visiting by general practitioners in England and Wales. BMJ. 1996;313:207–10.
6. Kao H, Conant R, Soriano T, McCormick W. The past, present and future of house calls. Clin Geriatr Med. 2009;25(1):19–34.
7. Steel RK, Muliner M, Boling PA. Medical schools and home care. N Engl J Med. 1994;331:1098–9.
8. Ornstein KA, Leff B, Kovinsky KE, et al. Epidemiology of the homebound population in the US. JAMA Intern Med. 2015;175(7):1180–6.
9. Leff B, Burton JR. The future history of home care and physician house calls in the United States. J Gerontol. 2001;56A:M603–8.
10. CMS Press Release June 18, 2015: Affordable Care Act payment model saves more than $25 million in first performance year. https://www.cms.gov/Newsroom/MediaReleaseDatabase/Press-releases/2015-Press-releases-items/2015-06-18.html.
11. Unwin BK, Tatum PE. House calls. Am Fam Physician. 2011;83(8):925–31.
12. CMS Manual System. Pub 100-02 Medicare Benefit Policy: Transmittal 192. Change Request 8818. Department of Health & Human Services (DHHS). Centers for Medicare & Medicaid

Services (CMS). 21 Aug 2014. http://www.cms.gov/Regulations-and-Guidance/Guidance/Transmittals/downloads/R192BP.pdf. Accessed 19 July 2015.

13. Occupational Safety & Health Administration. Safety and health topics: home healthcare. https://www.osha.gov/SLTC/home_healthcare. Accessed 19 July 2015.

14. American Medical Association Home Care Advisory Panel. Guidelines for the medical management of the home-care patient. Arch Fam Med. 1993;2:194–206.

15. Etchells E. Community tools: Aid to Capacity Evaluation (ACE). University of Toronto Joint Centre for Bioethics. http://www.jcb.utoronto.ca/tools/ace_download.shtml. Accessed 20 July 2015.

Aging in Place: Selecting and Supporting Caregivers of the Older Adult

8

Jennifer Fernandez, Jennifer Reckrey, and Lee Ann Lindquist

The population of adults aged 65 and older is expanding rapidly, and about 30 % have functional or cognitive limitations [1–3], 30 % have mobility limitations [4], and 20 % have chronic disabilities [5]. These limitations and disabilities often manifest themselves as problems in independently completing activities of daily living (ADLs) (feeding, mobility, transfers, toileting, dressing, grooming, bathing) and instrumental activities of daily living (iADLs) (cooking, cleaning, laundry, shopping phone, transportation, medications). Faced with these limitations yet wishing to stay in their homes as long as possible, many elders seek support from family, friends, or hired caregivers [6].

Most research literature categorizes caregivers as either "informal" or "formal." An "informal" caregiver is defined as any relative, partner, friend, or neighbor who has a significant personal relationship with, and provides a broad range of assistance for, an older person or an adult with a chronic or disabling condition [7]. Another term used to describe an informal caregiver is the family or unpaid caregiver, and for the purposes of this chapter, we will refer to them as such. Family caregivers are often family and friends who voluntarily assist individuals with their ADL and iADL needs. While there are some state-run programs that provide funding to family members and friends who provide this care, most unpaid caregivers receive no compensation for the care they provide. These individuals may be primary or secondary caregivers and may live with or separately from the person

J. Fernandez • L.A. Lindquist
Division of General Internal Medicine and Geriatrics, Northwestern University Feinberg
School of Medicine, 750 N. Lake Shore Drive, 10th Floor, Chicago, IL 60611, USA
e-mail: jennifer.fernandez@northwestern.edu; LAL425@md.northwestern.edu

J. Reckrey (✉)
Departments of Medicine and Geriatrics and Palliative Medicine, Icahn School of Medicine
at Mount Sinai, One Gustave L. Levy Place Box 1253, New York, NY 10029, USA
e-mail: Jennifer.reckrey@mountsinai.org

© Springer International Publishing Switzerland 2016
L.A. Lindquist (ed.), *New Directions in Geriatric Medicine*,
DOI 10.1007/978-3-319-28137-7_8

receiving care. "Formal" caregivers are caregivers associated with a formal service system [7]. In practice, these caregivers are referred to as "paid" caregivers, and for the purposes of this chapter, we will refer to them as such. Paid caregivers assist individuals with their ADL and iADL needs within a person's place of residence, in outdoor environments, or both. Paid caregivers are also called home care aides, personal care attendants, personal care assistants, direct care workers, private duty attendants, personal companions, sitters, or homemakers [8]. In contrast to certified nursing assistants or nurses, paid caregivers do not receive standardized patient care training.

As primary care providers care for the growing elderly population, they will routinely encounter both paid and family caregivers in their practices. The objectives of this chapter are to:

1. Review key background information about family and paid caregivers that will help providers better understand their role and the challenges they may encounter
2. Discuss the benefits of family caregiving
3. Discuss caregiver stress and the burden of family caregiving, review ways to screen for caregiver stress, and discuss how these issues can be addressed in primary care
4. List resources for caregivers
5. Discuss considerations when hiring paid caregivers
6. Review best practices for engaging paid caregivers

Family Caregivers

Background

More than 34 million family caregivers care for adults who are ill or have disabilities [9]. The average family caregiver is female, between the ages of 46 and 49, and the majority provides care for a relative (85 %), while one in ten provides care for a spouse [10]. Most caregivers have been in their role for 4 years [10]. Roughly half of care recipients live in their own home (48 %). However, as hours of care increase, so do the chances that the care recipient co-resides with the caregiver [10].

Family caregivers spend an average of 24.4 h/week providing care, and when asked the main reason their recipient needs care, "old age" (14 %), dementia (8 %), and surgery/wounds (8 %) are the most cited reasons [10]. Other common conditions that family caregivers provide care for include cancer (7 %), mobility (7 %), and mental/emotional health issues (5 %) [10]. Family caregivers provide an estimated 90 % of the long-term care needed by elderly and disabled individuals in the community [11].While most family caregivers assist patients with their activities of daily living (ADLs) and instrumental activities of daily living (IADLs), recent studies have shown that these mostly nonmedical caregivers are increasingly performing nursing tasks such as injections, tube feedings, and catheter and colostomy care [12]. In one study, 14 % of family caregivers find these tasks difficult, and most (42 %) are performing them without any formal training or preparation [12].

While we often think of the direct cost of paid caregivers, the economic impact of family caregivers is large. In 2007, it was estimated that it would cost $375 billion to replace the care provided by family caregivers with paid services. This is up from an estimated $350 billion in 2006 [9, 13]. However, providing care comes at a cost to the caregiver as well. In 2007, it was reported that family caregivers spent an average of $5531 out of pocket [9] and about 37 % of caregivers for someone age 50 and older reduced their work hours or quit their job in 2007 [13].

Caregiver Burden and Benefits of Caregiving

Providing care to a disabled loved one can result in a burden that impacts the emotional, physical, and economic health of the caregivers. Caregiver burden has been defined as a multidimensional response to the negative appraisal and perceived stress resulting from taking care of an ill individual [14]. Caregiver burden is often exhibited as psychological distress (depression, anxiety) or physical health problems (impaired immune response, health risk behaviors). Caregivers frequently suffer from depression, exhibit maladaptive coping strategies, and express concern about their poor quality of life [15–17]. They also report more physical and psychological symptoms and use more frequent prescription medications and healthcare services than comparable non-caregivers [17–19]. Caring for a close relative (spouse or parent) has been shown to be more emotionally stressful than caring for another relative or nonrelative [10], and being in a primary caregiving role is an independent risk factor for increasing mortality in the caregiver [20].

Caregiver burden has many social and economic consequences for the caregiver. It can lead to a loss or reduction in employment [21], decreased quality in childcare [22, 23], and marital conflict [24]. One in five caregivers reports financial strain/stress, and this is noted to be greater among co-resident caregivers [10]. Caregiver burden may also impact the patients who receive care, and caregiver burden has been associated with hospitalization, paid home care use, and nursing home placement [6, 25–29].

It may be particularly important for primary care providers to be aware of a new demographic known as the "sandwich generation," people who care for their dependent children while supporting their aging parents. Just over one out of every eight Americans aged 40 to 60 is both raising a child and caring for a parent. In addition, between seven to ten million adults are caring for their aging parents from a long distance (Pew Research Center). Sandwich caregivers often try to balance child and parent care with their own full-time work and may be particularly overworked and isolated. They may feel that they are not able to fully perform any of their roles well. Subsequently, sandwich caregivers are at an increased risk for developing depression, stress, burnout, anxiety, and poor self-care.

It is important that primary care providers screen for caregiver burden in the family caregivers who keep their patients functioning in the community. There are tools that have been developed to evaluate for caregiver burden: Caregiver Stress Index,

Table 8.1 Suggested questions for assessing caregiver burden during an office visit [31]

Screening question	Area of concern
Do you feel that you are currently under a lot of stress? What aspects of your day are the most stressful?	Mental health
Have you been feeling down or blue lately?	Mental health
Have you been feeling more anxious and irritable lately?	Mental health
Do your family and friends visit often? Do they telephone often?	Social support
Do your friends and family watch your relative for you so that you have time for yourself?	Social support
Do you have any outside help?	Resources
Is your relative with dementia having any behaviors, such as wandering, that are difficult to manage?	Behavioral management
What do you do to relieve your stress and tension?	Coping

Caregiver Burden Inventory, Caregiver Reaction Assessment, Caregiving Outcomes Scale, etc. The Caregiver Stress Index and the Caregiver Reaction Assessment are self-reported questionnaires that assess caregiver burden [30]. The Caregiver Burden Inventory is a self-reported 29-item questionnaire that includes questions on the caregiver's health, psychological well-being, finances, social life, and the relationship between the caregiver and patient. It is one of the tools used most consistently in research studies [30]. The Caregiving Outcomes Scale is a brief 10-item screening tool that uses a 7-point Likert scale [30]. While many of the available screening tools are used routinely in a research context, simply asking the caregiver a few questions during the office visit is also a good way to help primary care providers identify burdened caregivers (Table 8.1).

Another resource to screen for caregiver burden is the Caregiver Stress Checklist, available through the Alzheimer's Association webpage. The eight-step simple checklist screens for caregiver stress and then links the caregiver to tips for managing stress, provides information about respite care, and provides community support groups and online connections to support [32].

Rewards of Family Caregiving

While it is important to recognize caregiver burden, it is also important to remember that there are benefits of caregiving. The benefit of family caregivers for patients is clear. Studies have shown that family caregiver support often delays or prevents long-term care use and that patients with family caregivers tend to have shorter hospital stays [33, 34]. Conversely, the absence of family support has been linked to hospital readmissions [35]. However, family caregiving often provides benefits to the caregiver as well. Family caregivers often experience a feeling of duty accomplished, self-satisfaction, and reciprocity [36]. If they co-reside with the care recipient, they can often share the cost of living and reduce travel time [2].

Avoiding Caregiver Burnout

Resources for Family Caregivers

Many caregiver associations and organizations provide assistance for caregivers. One is the National Family Caregiver Support Program (NFCSP), which provides grants to fund a range of supports that assist family and other unpaid caregivers to care for their loved ones at home for as long as possible. The NFCSP provides five types of services to support informal caregivers: information to caregivers about available services, assistance to caregivers in gaining access to those services, individual counseling, organization of support groups, and on a limited basis caregiver training, respite care, and supplemental services (ACL). However, the services provided by the NFCSP vary widely from state to state, and this leaves gaps in many areas [37]. Other caregiver resources include the AARP Caregiving website, American Red Cross Family Caregiver Program, Family Caregiver Alliance, Administration on Aging, and Elderly Healthcare Organization [38]. In addition, disease-specific support groups like Alzheimer's Association often provide support and resources for caregivers.

Respite Services

Another important resource for caregivers is respite services. Respite care is the provision of short-term accommodation in a facility outside the home in which a loved one may be placed [39]. Respite services provide short-term breaks for caregivers that can help relieve stress, but caregivers are often unaware that respite services exist and need to be informed about them by their primary care provider. Respite care services have been shown to both benefit patients and caregivers. Studies have found that respite care services for the elderly with chronic disabilities resulted in fewer hospital admissions for acute medical care [40] and that as the use of respite care increased, the probability of nursing home placement decreased [41]. Respite care has been shown to decrease caregiver-related stress in those using adult day care and improve psychological well-being in both short- (3 months) and long-term use (12 months) [42].

Job Assistance

Finally, family caregivers who are also working paying jobs as full-time or part-time employees may find support in their workplace. Employers may offer resource/referral services, flexible scheduling, dependent care assistance plans (DCAPs), and family care leave of absences [43]. Referral services and flexible scheduling vary from employer to employer. Dependent care assistance plans allow employees to take a pretax deduction of up to $5000 annually for a single person or married couple filing a joint income tax return or $2500 annually for each married participant who files a separate income tax return. To qualify, either the caregiver or spouse must care for someone who is a dependent (or would be a dependent were it not for certain described circumstances) who lives with them. The Family and Medical Leave Act (FLMA) allows employees who have been employed for 12 months and who work in places with at least 50 employees or who work in public agencies or public and private elementary and secondary school to take unpaid, job-protected leave for up to 12 weeks/year for specified family and medical reasons[44]. As companies see declines in productivity because of competing demands from caregiving, hopefully they will increase assistance to their employees who also provide unpaid care to loved ones.

Paid Caregivers

While the vast majority of the nearly $120 billion spent on long-term care services is spent on residential care, the amount spent on paid caregivers has increased over the past 25 years [45]. About 90 % of paid caregivers are women and 16.2 % are not US citizens [10], 31.5 % have not graduated from high school, and only 46 % are able to secure full-time work all year round [10]. As they care for elderly, frail patients, paid caregivers are often vulnerable and isolated themselves: one study found that 63 % were born outside the USA and over 50 % had no family support in the USA [46].

Paid caregivers perform a wide variety of tasks in the home including meal preparation, household chores, garbage removal, dressing, bathing, toileting, medication reminding, and following physician instructions [46]. Medication reminding in particular can be a complicated task especially when the care recipient is an older adult with multiple medical problems and uses over 15 medications administered at varying frequencies. A recent study demonstrated that 36 % of paid caregivers, hired privately or through an agency, were found to have limited health literacy and that 60 % of caregivers made errors when they were asked to read and interpret medication labels [46].

Paid caregiver wages are low, and paid caregivers on average earn 8–9 dollars an hour [46–48]. Paid caregivers have historically been exempt from federal minimum wage and hour protection laws since what was known as the "companionship exemption" as initiated in 1974, but recent federal legislation has now narrowed the definition of companionship services and employers such as home care agencies can no longer claim exemptions from labor protection laws [49].

While Medicare-funded organizations like skilled nursing facilities and Medicare-certified home health agencies must conform to training standards which include 75 h of federally mandated training for direct care workers, most home care workers are not paid through Medicare [50]. Individual states determine training and supervision requirements for paid caregivers, and these standards vary tremendously from state to state. For example, only 29 states require a license for home care provider agencies, and of these 29 states, 26 require an orientation (when specified, the duration ranged from 8 to 60 h), but only 16 states specified what that orientation should include [50].

Hiring a Paid Caregiver

While some paid caregivers are hired through Medicaid programs, many patients and families are in the position of privately hiring a caregiver. Paid caregivers can be hired through (1) caregiver placement services, (2) caregiver agencies, or (3) directly through contracting with the caregiver. Caregiver placement services exist in some but not all states. These services charge a fee to connect patients and families with caregivers; the services do not provide any additional caregiver training or support and patients and families pay caregivers directly.

It is more common for patients or families to hire paid caregivers by either contracting with agency or contracting directly with a caregiver. Both of these approaches have pros and cons that are described (Table 8.2), and primary care providers may be asked to help patients and families weigh these options. It is also important to advise families that they do not have to settle on the paid caregiver they are initially assigned. People innately may not blend with their caregivers on a personal, cultural, or emotional level. It is acceptable to ask for replacement caregivers or interview/trial other caregivers until the right fit is found.

In addition, patients and families should be aware of the variability in the quality of agencies providing home care and how they hire, train, and supervise caregivers. In hiring, many agencies required prior "life experiences" (68.8 %) but few of which (27.2 %) were specific to caregiving. Screening measures may include federal criminal background checks (55.8 %) and drug testing (31.8 %). General caregiver training length ranged from 0 to 7 days. Supervision ranged from none to weekly and included home visits, telephone calls, and caregivers visiting the central office. While most agencies stated that the paid caregiver could perform

Table 8.2 Pros and cons of direct and agency hiring

Pros of direct hiring	Cons of direct hiring
Comfort in knowing the caregiver or having the caregiver vouched for by another	Background check needs to be done by hiring person
Less costly than other options (e.g., agencies)	Lack of backup caregivers if caregiver is not able to be present
Able to directly assign tasks and provide feedback to caregivers	Caregiver may not have health insurance; may need to pay for health insurance
	Will have to perform supervision of caregiver directly
Pros of hiring through a caregiver agency	Cons of hiring through a caregiver agency
Caregiver employees have been vetted by the agency	Vetting process for caregivers may be variable by different agencies
Availability of backup caregivers if caregiver is not able to be present	Costs may be higher than other means of hiring
Supervision to be expected through the caregiver agency	Supervision may vary by different agencies
Training to be expected through the caregiver agency	Training may vary by different agencies

Table 8.3 Questions to ask when using an agency to hire a caregiver

1. What recruiting methods are used?
2. What are the hiring requirements?
3. What type of screenings is performed on caregivers before they are hired?
4. Are the caregivers insured and bonded through the agency?
5. How does the agency assess what the caregiver is capable of doing?
6. Does the agency train caregivers? What does that training entail? What type of health-related training do the caregivers have (CPR)?
7. What is the substitution policy if the regular caregiver is not available?
8. If you are not satisfied with a particular caregiver, will the agency replace the person "without cause"?
9. Does the agency provide a supervisor to evaluate the quality of home care on a regular basis? How frequently? And is it in person or over the phone?
10. What competencies are expected of the caregivers you send to the home?

skills such as medication reminding (96.0 %), skill competency was assessed only according to caregiver self-report (58.5 %), testing (35.2 %), and client feedback (35.2 %) [51].

It is important for primary care providers to recommend that if patients and families use agencies to hire caregivers, they should carefully vet the agency that they select. Existing recommendations outline what patients and families should ask a caregiver agency that they are considering working with (Table 8.3). While these may not be all encompassing, they are a start in identifying a fair and quality agency. The Home Care Association of America (HCAOA) is an association of private duty home care providers, and patients and families can use their website http://www.hcaoa.org/ to connect with home care agencies in their area (Table 8.3).

Incorporating the Caregiver in the Healthcare Encounter

It is paramount that primary care providers ask their patients if they have a caregiver. If families are planning to hire a caregiver, recommending training on medication administration is reasonable [52]. If families already have a formal caregiver, the caregiver must be included when medication instructions are given. The Teach-Back method is extremely useful for low-health literacy patients and caregivers. The Teach-Back method is a communication confirmation method used to confirm whether a patient or caregiver understands what is being explained to them. If a patient or caregiver understands, they are able to "teach back" the information accurately. When available, services that help patients with setting up pillboxes are also excellent resources for patients and caregivers [53]. Primary care providers should also ask caregivers about self-care and personal wellness and monitor for signs of depression/suicidality in caregivers.

While most caregivers are motivated to help older adults, there are examples in the lay press where caregivers have diverted patients' medications for personal habits or financial gain. While this is unfortunate and not typical, prescription medication diversion by caregivers does occur. If an older adult patient is experiencing uncontrolled pain while on large doses of medications or is losing medications and requesting frequent refills, primary care providers should consider if caregivers are diverting patient prescriptions.

The health of the caregiver is also an important factor to consider when treating the older adult patient. With the population aging, more older adults are reaching their 90s and 100s. These super-agers frequently have caregivers involved in their daily lives. When patients are over 90 years old, family caregivers are often older adults themselves, sometimes in the age range of 70–80 years. If caregivers are experiencing cognitive decline themselves while providing medication reminders or other essential care, the older adult may be in peril. If a caregiver is hospitalized, an emergency plan needs to be placed and the clinician should inquire about this plan. In addition, the primary care provider needs to be aware of the factors that may affect the health of a caregiver and therefore may jeopardize the health of the older adult. In particular, there are many paid caregivers who do not receive healthcare due to immigration status, financial hardship, or other personal issues. Asking about the caregiver's health and how they are doing can be easily integrated into the cordial greeting or conversation in any office encounter. Further, offering caregivers the opportunity to receive a health assessment, receive vaccines, or connect to healthcare enrollment can make a large impact on both the caregiver and the care that the older adult receives.

Summary

The number of caregivers is likely to increase as our growing population of older adults ages in place. Understanding the issues affecting caregivers, both familial and paid, is essential for clinicians who provide care to older adults. Recognizing an overburdened caregiver and providing information on opportunities for relief can dramatically improve the care of older adult patients. It takes a team of people to care for the older adult patient, and incorporating caregivers into the healthcare team is vital.

Key Points
1. Older adults who have functional or cognitive limitations depend on support from two main types of caregivers: (1) family or informal caregivers and (2) paid or formal caregivers.
2. Assessing burden and the health of the caregiver is important to maintain the health of the older adult.
3. To alleviate burden in family caregivers, clinicians can offer information on respite services, area resources, or the option of hiring a paid caregiver to supplement care.
4. Hiring a paid caregiver can be accomplished through thoughtful vetting and asking key questions, which are provided.

5. The pros and cons of hiring a paid caregiver through an agency versus direct hiring should be considered.
6. Incorporating the caregiver into the healthcare encounter is integral in ensuring that the older adult receives optimal care.

References

1. U.S. Department of Health and Human Services. Administration on Aging (AOA). 2015. http://www.aoa.acl.gov/Aging_Statistics/index.aspx. Cited 8 Aug 2015.
2. Pezzin LE, Pollak RA, Schone BS. Bargaining power, parental caregiving, and intergenerational coresidence. J Gerontol B Psychol Sci Soc Sci. 2015;70(6):969–80. Epub 2014 Jul 3.
3. Congressional Budget Office. Rising demand for long-term services and supports for elderly people. June 2013, 113th congress. Pub. No. 4240:1–44.
4. Freedman VA, Martin LG. Understanding trends in functional limitations among older Americans. Am J Public Health. 1998;88(10):1457–62.
5. Manton KG, Gu X. Changes in the prevalence of chronic disability in the United States black and nonblack population above age 65 from 1982 to 1999. Proc Natl Acad Sci U S A. 2001;98(11):6354–9.
6. Yaffe K, et al. Patient and caregiver characteristics and nursing home placement in patients with dementia. JAMA. 2002;287(16):2090–7.
7. Caregiving F.C.A-N.C.o. Definitions. 2015. https://caregiver.org/definitions-0. Cited 26 Aug 2015
8. Lindquist LA, et al. Paid caregiver motivation, work conditions, and falls among senior clients. Arch Gerontol Geriatr. 2012;55(2):442–5.
9. Ari N, Houser MJG. Valuing the invaluable: the economic value of family caregiving. 2008. http://www.aarp.org/relationships/caregiving/info-11-2008/i13_caregiving.html. Cited 14 Aug 2015.
10. National Alliance for Caregiving. Caregiving in the U.S 2015. 2015. http://www.caregiving.org/caregiving2015/. Cited 14 Aug 2015.
11. IOM. Retooling for an aging America: building the health care workforce. 2008. http://www.nap.edu/catalog/12089/retooling-for-an-aging-america-building-the-health-care-workforce. Cited 14 Aug 2015
12. Reinhard SC, Samis S. Home alone: family caregivers providing complex chronic care. 2012. http://www.aarp.org/home-family/caregiving/info-10-2012/home-alone-family-caregivers-providing-complex-chronic-care.html. Cited 14 Aug 2015.
13. Gibson MJ, Houser A. Valuing the invaluable: a new look at the economic value of family caregiving. Issue Brief (Public Policy Inst (Am Assoc Retired Pers)). 2007;IB82:1–12.
14. Kim H, et al. Predictors of caregiver burden in caregivers of individuals with dementia. J Adv Nurs. 2012;68(4):846–55.
15. Molyneux GJ, et al. Prevalence and predictors of carer burden and depression in carers of patients referred to an old age psychiatric service. Int Psychogeriatr. 2008;20(6):1193–202.
16. Papastavrou E, et al. Caring for a relative with dementia: family caregiver burden. J Adv Nurs. 2007;58(5):446–57.
17. Serrano-Aguilar PG, Lopez-Bastida J, Yanes-Lopez V. Impact on health-related quality of life and perceived burden of informal caregivers of individuals with Alzheimer's disease. Neuroepidemiology. 2006;27(3):136–42.
18. Brodaty H, Green A. Defining the role of the caregiver in Alzheimer's disease treatment. Drugs Aging. 2002;19(12):891–8.
19. Schulz R, Martire LM. Family caregiving of persons with dementia: prevalence, health effects, and support strategies. Am J Geriatr Psychiatry. 2004;12(3):240–9.

20. Schulz R, Beach SR. Caregiving as a risk factor for mortality: the Caregiver Health Effects Study. JAMA. 1999;282(23):2215–9.
21. Scharlach AE. Caregiving and employment: competing or complementary roles? Gerontologist. 1994;34(3):378–85.
22. Chassin L, et al. The association between membership in the sandwich generation and health behaviors: a longitudinal study. J Appl Dev Psychol. 2010;31(1):38–46.
23. Rogerson PA, Kim D. Population distribution and redistribution of the baby-boom cohort in the United States: recent trends and implications. Proc Natl Acad Sci U S A. 2005;102(43):15319–24.
24. Brody EM, et al. Differential effects of daughters' marital status on their parent care experiences. Gerontologist. 1992;32(1):58–67.
25. Bookwala J, et al. Concurrent and long-term predictors of older adults' use of community-based long-term care services: the Caregiver Health Effects Study. J Aging Health. 2004;16(1):88–115.
26. Gaugler JE, et al. Caregiving and institutionalization of cognitively impaired older people: utilizing dynamic predictors of change. Gerontologist. 2003;43(2):219–29.
27. Kuzuya M, et al. Impact of caregiver burden on adverse health outcomes in community-dwelling dependent older care recipients. Am J Geriatr Psychiatry. 2011;19(4):382–91.
28. Miller EA, Rosenheck RA, Schneider LS. Caregiver burden, health utilities, and institutional service use in Alzheimer's disease. Int J Geriatr Psychiatry. 2012;27(4):382–93.
29. Nakagawa Y, Nasu S. Association between components of family caregivers' sense of burden and types of paid care services provided in Japan. Aging Ment Health. 2011;15(6):687–701.
30. Deeken JF, et al. Care for the caregivers: a review of self-report instruments developed to measure the burden, needs, and quality of life of informal caregivers. J Pain Symptom Manage. 2003;26(4):922–53.
31. Parks SM, Novielli KD. A practical guide to caring for caregivers. Am Fam Physician. 2000;62(12):2613–22.
32. Association A. Caregiver stress check. http://www.alz.org/care/alzheimers-dementia-stress-check.asp. Cited 26 Aug 2015.
33. Mittelman MS, et al. Improving caregiver well-being delays nursing home placement of patients with Alzheimer disease. Neurology. 2006;67(9):1592–9.
34. Spillman BC, Long SK. Does high caregiver stress lead to nursing home entry? 2007. http://aspe.hhs.gov/basic-report/does-high-caregiver-stress-lead-nursing-home-entry. Cited 18 Aug 2015.
35. Picone G, Mark Wilson R, Chou SY. Analysis of hospital length of stay and discharge destination using hazard functions with unmeasured heterogeneity. Health Econ. 2003;12(12):1021–34.
36. Nardi Ede F, Sawada NO, Santos JL. The association between the functional incapacity of the older adult and the family caregiver's burden. Rev Lat Am Enfermagem. 2013;21(5):1096–103.
37. Thai JN, Barnhart CE, Cagle J, Smith AK. It just consumes your life: quality of life for informal caregivers of diverse older adults with late-life disability. Am J Hosp Palliat Care. 2015 May 6.
38. Prevention C.f.D.C.a. Caregiving resources. http://www.cdc.gov/aging/caregiving/resources.htm. Cited 26 Aug 2015.
39. Force NRCT. Benefits and cost-saving due to respite. http://archrespite.org/docs/Cost_Fact_Sheet_11-09.pdf. Cited 30 Aug 2015.
40. Chang JI, et al. Patient outcomes in hospital-based respite: a study of potential risks and benefits. J Am Board Fam Pract. 1992;5(5):475–81.
41. Kosloski K, Montgomery RJ. The impact of respite use on nursing home placement. Gerontologist. 1995;35(1):67–74.
42. Zarit SH, et al. Stress reduction for family caregivers: effects of adult day care use. J Gerontol B Psychol Sci Soc Sci. 1998;53(5):S267–77.
43. Seaward MR. The sandwich generation copes with elder care. Benefits Q. 1999;15(2):41–8.

44. Labor UDO. Family and medical leave. 2015. http://www.dol.gov/dol/topic/benefits-leave/fmla.htm. Cited 30 Aug 2015.
45. Kaye HS, Harrington C, LaPlante MP. Long-term care: who gets it, who provides it, who pays, and how much? Health Aff (Millwood). 2010;29(1):11–21.
46. Lindquist LA, et al. Inadequate health literacy among paid caregivers of seniors. J Gen Intern Med. 2011;26(5):474–9.
47. Institute T.A. Reinventing low wage work ideas that can work for employees, employers and the economy. http://www.aspenwsi.org/wordpress/wp-content/uploads/Profiles-of-the-Direct-Care-Workforce-and-PHI.pdf. Cited 18 Aug 2015.
48. MetLife. Market survey of long-term care costs. 2012. https://www.metlife.com/assets/cao/mmi/publications/studies/2012/studies/mmi-2012-market-survey-long-term-care-costs.pdf. Cited 18 Aug 2015.
49. Facts F. Understanding the revised companionship exemption. 2013. Understanding the Revised Companionship Exemption. Cited 18 Aug 2015.
50. Kelly CM, Morgan JC, Jason KJ. Home care workers: interstate differences in training requirements and their implications for quality. J Appl Gerontol. 2013;32(7):804–32.
51. Lindquist LA, Cameron KA, Messerges-Bernstein J, Friesema E, Zickuhr L, Baker DW, Wolf M. Hiring and screening practices of agencies supplying paid caregivers to older adults. J Am Geriatr Soc. 2012;60:1253–9.
52. Sudore RL, Covinsky KE. Respecting elders by respecting their paid caregivers. J Gen Intern Med. 2011;26(5):464–5.
53. Paasche-Orlow MK, et al. The prevalence of limited health literacy. J Gen Intern Med. 2005;20(2):175–84.

Skilled Nursing Facilities and Post-hospitalization Options for Older Adults

Jill Huded and Fernanda Heitor

When hospitalized, older individuals are vulnerable to delirium, adverse drug reactions, pressure ulcers, bladder and bowel dysfunction, dehydration, malnutrition, and functional decline. These hazards of hospitalization are associated with long recovery times and frequently contribute to the need to transition to post-acute care facilities for rehabilitation and ongoing complex care.

Care transitions are common in older adults. In the 6 months following a hip fracture, patients experience an average of 3.5 relocations between home, hospital, rehabilitation, and nursing facilities [1]. There may be more than seven handoffs amongst physicians during one hospital stay alone, not including post-hospitalization transfers [2]. Excellent care transitions require comprehensive discharge planning, which should ideally begin at hospital admission. At patient admission, a process should be initiated to ascertain future functional, rehabilitative, nursing, and medical needs that will be required by the older adult at time of discharge. This typically requires the input of physicians, social workers, physical and occupational therapists, and nursing staff.

Clinicians must have a general understanding of post-acute care options to adequately guide patient and families through the process of discharge planning. Increased education and exposure during training about SNFs will likely improve care transitions [3]. The role of the clinician in the transition process includes understanding patients' underlying illness, prognoses, and functional limitations;

J. Huded (✉)
Department of Medicine, Louis Stokes Cleveland Veterans Affairs Medical Center, Case
Western Reserve University School of Medicine, 10701 East Boulevard,
Cleveland, OH 44106, USA
e-mail: jill.huded@va.gov

F. Heitor
Division of General Internal Medicine and Geriatrics, Northwestern University Feinberg
School of Medicine, 675 North St. Clair Street, Suite 18-200, Galter,
Chicago, IL 60611, USA
e-mail: Fernanda.Heitor@Northwestern.edu

© Springer International Publishing Switzerland 2016
L.A. Lindquist (ed.), *New Directions in Geriatric Medicine*,
DOI 10.1007/978-3-319-28137-7_9

facilitating thoughtful family and patient discussions; appreciating the significance of caregiver burden; having an awareness of elder abuse; and ensuring a thorough handoff [4]. Communication with health-care staff at the next transition site by physicians has been shown to decrease future emergency department visits and promote treatment in line with patients' goals of care [5].

Post-hospitalization discharge destinations that will be discussed within this chapter include:

- Acute inpatient rehabilitation
- Long-term acute care hospital (LTACH)
- Subacute rehabilitation (skilled nursing facility—SNF)
- Long-term care (nursing home)
- Independent and assisted living facilities
- Continuing care retirement community (CCRC)
- Home health (skilled and unskilled)
- Adult day care
- Hospice care

Determining the Discharge Needs of the Patient and Family

The first task when selecting a post-acute facility is determining the type of care the resident will need. Care needs are determined by activities of daily living (ADLs), independent activities of daily living (IADLs), cognition, and mobility. These domains are assessed by physicians, physical and occupational therapists, and care teams through well-validated scales and screens. ADLs such as bathing, dressing, feeding, and toileting are measured with the Katz ADL scale [6] and Barthel scale [7]. IADLs of cooking, cleaning, managing finances, transportation, medications, and using the telephone are assessed with the Lawton IADL scale [8]. The MMSE [9], MoCA [10], Mini-Cog [11], and CAM [12] are used to evaluate cognition and delirium. Mobility can be assessed with the Timed Up and Go Test [13] in the clinic or by PT and OT. Once the above care needs, in addition to acute medical needs such as IV antibiotics or wound care, are established, facilities that meet these needs based on qualifying diagnoses, nursing staff, and/or therapy availability can further be pursued.

Resources for Selecting the Post-hospitalization Care Facility

After the type of facility is determined, options can be narrowed down based on location, philosophy, religious affiliation (if any), and policies. Inpatient and outpatient social workers, discharge planners, and home health agencies will guide patients and families through the selection process by providing a list of appropriate facilities in the desired geographic region. The quality of all Medicare- and Medicaid-certified vendors in the USA can be found at Nursing Home Compare, an online quality report provided by the Centers for Medicare and Medicaid Services. Information can be found by searching for facilities by location or name at http:// www.medicare.gov/nursinghomecompare/. A 5-star rating system incorporates health inspections, quality measures, and staffing into an overall score. Data from on-site health inspections and information from the Minimum Data Set (MDS) are reported and updated once monthly (see below) [14].

Eldercare Locator is another source of information about local services. Its mission is to connect older adults and their families with trustworthy community resources, such as transportation and meals, and provide caregivers with training or respite. Eldercare partners with the National Association of Area Agencies on Aging and can be contacted by calling 1-800-677-1116 or visiting eldercare.gov.

Aging and Disability Resource Centers (ADRC) partner with the Administration for Community Living and Centers for Medicare and Medicaid Services to optimize care transitions, provide long-term care counseling, and streamline access to support services for older individuals and those with disabilities. ADRC assists seniors with Medicaid financial applications and is committed to helping individuals make informed decisions and coordinate care for all levels of financial resources. ADRC partners with hospitals, nursing facilities, and rehabilitation institutions in developing care-transition programs. All states are now providing ADRC services. Information can be found at adrc-tae.acl.gov.

When researching long-term care living options, such as assisted living and nursing homes, local long-term care ombudsmen can provide assistance. More than 8000 volunteers and 1000 paid staff work in state ombudsman program supported by the Administration on Aging. They provide general information on nursing homes, investigate complaints about specific facilities, and make site visits each year. The Eldercare Locator (1-800-677-1116) can provide contact information for your local ombudsmen or you can visit ltcombudsman.org.

Questions for patients and families to address when selecting a care facility
1. What care does the patient require?
What acute and chronic medical needs does the patient have?
Do they need wound care or IV medications?
Are there functional mobility needs?
Do they need assistance with bathing, dressing, feeding, or toileting?
Do they have cognitive impairment or confusion?
Do they have difficulty swallowing or speaking and have speech therapy needs?
Do they need help with medications?
Are their needs not met by the current caregiver?
What are their personal goals of care and view on end-of-life care?
Are care needs likely to escalate over several years, suggesting a Continuing Care Retirement Community (CCRC) would be appropriate?
2. What is the best vendor?
Ideally, the patient or a family member will visit the facility
Where is the facility located? Is it important to be near family or friends?
Is it affiliated with a religious or cultural organization?

(continued)

(continued)

Questions for patients and families to address when selecting a care facility
How much will it cost after third-party payers are accounted for?
Is there current bed availability?
How is the facility's overall rating? Health inspection? Staffing? Quality measures?
Ask about the vendor's strengths and weakness
See www.medicare.gov/nursinghomecompare/search.html
Who develops and has input into the care plan?
Who are the doctors that will visit; when do they visit?
How does staff handle agitation, confusion, or other difficult behavior?
Is there consistency in staffing?
How many residents are each certified nursing assistant (CNA) and nurse assigned to?
Is there licensed nursing staff 24 h/day?
Can I meet the social worker?
Is therapy provided every day, even on weekends?
Do podiatrists, ophthalmologists, audiologists, or psychologists visit the facility?
Is there an arrangement with a nearby hospital?
Is the vendor Medicare and/or Medicaid certified?
3. Other questions
Are there resident policies, such as smoking or alcohol restrictions?
What social and recreational activities are provided?
Does each resident have a private room?
Can visitors visit at any time?
Will personal belongings be safe?
What are the dietary options? Can outside food and drinks be brought in?
Will staff help residents eat and drink if needed?
Are transportation services to physicians' appointments provided?
Are there extra costs for services such as transportation, health aid, or hair care?
What are the procedures for leaving the building?
Can personal pets visit?
Will the resident have input into the timing of eating, sleeping, and bathing activities?
Can we ask current residents about their experience with the facility?
Will the resident be treated in a respectful way?

Description of Post-hospitalization Options

Acute Inpatient Rehabilitation

Individuals who have experienced a loss of function from illness or injury may be eligible for acute inpatient rehabilitation. Examples of appropriate diagnoses include amputations, brain or spinal cord injuries, other neurological disorders, orthopedic injuries, and deconditioning secondary to an acute illness. Individuals can be admitted to acute rehab from home, acute care hospitals, or other facilities.

Patients must be medically and psychologically stable and cognitively able to participate in 3 h of therapy each day for 5 days weekly. Two skilled rehabilitation needs are required, including physical, occupational, or speech therapy, with an expectation of improvement throughout their stay. In addition to therapy, activities of daily living, group activities, and family and friend participation are encouraged and emphasized. Members of the treatment team include physicians (typically physiatrists, as opposed to internists or geriatricians at SNFs), nurses certified in rehabilitation nursing (CRRN), physical therapists, occupational therapists, speech therapists, psychologists, and dieticians. Prosthetic and orthotic services are typically available. Extensive family and caregiver training is emphasized, in addition to transition planning prior to discharge. There is no requirement for a 3-day acute care admission before acute rehabilitation as opposed to subacute rehabilitation. Similar to long-term acute care (LTAC) facilities, acute inpatient rehabilitation can typically provide IV therapy, wound care, respiratory therapy, tracheostomy care, PEG tube care, laboratory services, and dialysis.

Long-Term Acute Care Hospital

Long-term acute care hospitals provide acute care needs to critically ill individuals for extended periods of time, with an anticipated duration of greater than 25 days for Medicare coverage. They can be freestanding facilities or a "hospital-within-hospital" model. Residents are medically complex with several current active medical conditions necessitating daily physician interaction. Such needs include pulmonary or tracheostomy care, ventilator management and weaning, dialysis, IV medications, or advanced wound care. The majority of patients are admitted to LTACHs after admission to the intensive care unit or a step-down unit.

Skilled Nursing Facility

Skilled nursing facility (SNF) care is appropriate for patients with need for a skilled service and 24/7 monitoring by medical staff. Skilled services include intravenous therapy, artificial nutrition and hydration, complex wound care, ostomy care or rehabilitation with physical therapy, occupational therapy, or speech therapy. Medicare-covered services also include a semiprivate room, meals, medical social services, medications, medical supplies and equipment used in the facility, dietary counseling, and ambulance transportation (when other transportation endangers health) to the nearest supplier or needed services that are not available at the SNF. Pharmaceutical, laboratory, and radiology services are available. Overall goals of skilled nursing include recovering from a recent illness or surgery, regaining functional independence, or providing acute medical care. Care plans are developed by an interprofessional team to determine what kind of services are needed, who should provide these services, what equipment is needed at the SNF and then at home, and how much time is required to achieve the stated goals. Physical and occupational therapy services are typically provided at least 5 days weekly if indicated. Physicians are required to see a patient within 72 h of admission and once weekly thereafter, unless an acute medical concern arises.

The first 20 days of skilled nursing care are fully covered Medicare, and partial coverage is provided for days 21–100 after a 3-night qualifying acute inpatient hospital stay. Per Medicare, days spent under observation services in the hospital and the day of discharge do not count toward inpatient days. Coverage for subacute services may stop earlier once the treatment goal is met or if the patient "plateaus" and no longer demonstrates improvement. After a patient leaves the SNF, coverage for future skilled nursing care depends on how many days have passed since discharge. If the break was more than 30 days, the patient will need a new 3-day hospital stay to qualify for additional SNF care. This new hospital stay does not need to be for the same condition that the patient was treated for during the prior stay. The individual will be able to receive skilled nursing care for the remaining of the 100 days under SNF benefits. If the break in the skilled care lasted for at least 60 days in a row, this would end the current benefit period and would start a new SNF benefit period, meaning that 100 days of coverage would again be available. The Centers for Medicare and Medicaid Services provides a helpful nursing home checklist in "Your Guide to Choosing a Nursing Home or Other Long-Term Care" available online at www.medicare.gov/Pubs/pdf/02174.pdf.

Long-Term Care and Nursing Homes

Long-term care (LTC) includes care at home (unpaid and paid) and community services such as adult day care, skilled nursing facilities, assisted living facilities, and hospice/respite care. Seventy percent of adults 65 years and older will use long-term care at some point during their lives, for an average of 2.8–3 years in duration. Thirty-five percent of adults will receive LTC in the nursing home setting. Women are more likely to use these resources as they live 5 years longer than men on average [15]. LTC facilities welcoming to the LGBT community and cognizant of their unique needs are now available. The most comprehensive long-term care is administered in nursing homes, where nursing care and 24 h supervision can be delivered. Medicare will not pay for unskilled assistance for activities of daily living; therefore, LTC in a nursing facility is paid either out of pocket, by a public insurance program (Medicaid and the Department of Veterans Affairs), or private insurance program. Medicaid is the largest provider of LTC services in the USA. If a person's income meets state eligibility requirements and has an income below a certain level, they may qualify for Medicaid coverage. Private health insurance will typically only cover short-term care such as subacute rehabilitation or will reimburse policyholders for a preselected number of days in LTC with a maximum reimbursement per day. Life insurance policies can sometimes be converted into LTC coverage by decreasing the reimbursement at death.

Custodial and non-skilled personal care, such as bathing, dressing, and toileting assistance, will be provided. Physician, skilled nursing, pharmaceutical, dietary, mental, and social services will be provided as needed. The assigned physician will see the resident every 30 days for the first 90 days after admission, followed by once every 60 days or more frequently for acute medical concerns. A 10-day grace period for late visits is accepted. The physician following them in the nursing facility typically assumes the role of their primary care physician. A plan of care will be prepared by the resident's family or POA, physician, and a registered nurse (RN), outlining the medical, nursing, mental, and social needs of the resident and how these needs will be met. This plan of care will be periodically reviewed and tailored to meet their current needs.

Independent Living and Assisted Living

Independent living (IL) communities provide housing designed specifically for seniors. Units can be apartments, condos, and freestanding homes. Low-income senior housing complexes are available through the US Department of Housing and Urban Development (HUD). Retirement communities and continuing care retirement communities are other providers of IL. Activities, amenities, and recreational centers are typically provided and allow for resident interaction and stimulation. Beauty and barber salons, meals, and housekeeping are typically available. If personal care assistance is required, this must be purchased separately. IL can be ideal for seniors struggling to maintain their home, find it difficult to leave their home due to mobility or transportation barriers, and who are socially isolated.

Since the 1970s when the institutionalization of aging seniors came into question, Dr. Keren Brown Wilson combined "the three Hs: health, housing, and hospitality" as the founder of the assisted living (AL) model and the first nationally recognized AL facility in Oregon [16]. Growing from privately owned establishments to corporately run businesses, AL is now the fastest-growing option for LTC. Assisted living facilities are intended for residents who need assistance with ADLs while living in a homelike setting providing more privacy and participation than a nursing home. They receive more supervision with daily care, medications and meals than at home, but will not have 24-h nursing support. Traditionally, AL units are apartments housed in a building or on a campus with other units providing other levels of care. More recently, AL can be provided in smaller-scale residential facilities such as residential care homes and personal care and board homes.

More than half of AL residents are at least 85 years old, and in general, they are functionally dependent upon others in one or more capacity. Almost 40 % require assistance with three or more activities of daily living. The average length stay is 22 months. Nationwide, almost 20 % receive AL care through Medicaid and 80 % through private pay (http://www.alfa.org/alfa/Assisted_Living_Information.asp). A 2015 Cost of Care Survey found the average cost of a private AL room was $43,200 compared to over $90,000 per year for a private nursing home room. Most seniors pay out of pocket of IL or AL costs, with a small minority receiving financial coverage through Medicaid waiver programs, long-term care insurance, or veteran's benefits.

Information on AL facilities, outreach, and advocacy can be found at the websites of Assisted Living Federation of America (ALFA, http://www.alfa.org/alfa/default.asp), CCAL—Advancing Person-Centered Living (http://www.ccal.org/about-ccal/), and the National Center for Assisted Living (http://www.ahcancal.org/ncal/Pages/index.aspx).

Continuing Care Retirement Community

Continuing care retirement communities (or CCRCs) offer several levels of care at the same campus and typically included independent living, assisted living, memory care, and short- and long-term skilled nursing. They are also known as life care communities. Typically, adults will join a CCRC while they are independent and remain there through the end of life. Residents can upgrade their nursing care and transition to different facilities, as needs change and more services are needed. For example, if a resident is admitted to the hospital and has a skilled nursing need upon discharge, they will be guaranteed a room to receive subacute nursing until they are stable for their previous unit. CCRCs are costly, typically requiring an entrance fee followed by maintenance fees (called a life care contract). Entrance fees range from $100,000 to $1 million, with monthly charges costing between $3000 and $5000 initially. CCRCs may also offer fee-for-service contracts, which have lower entrance and monthly fees but require market value payments if a higher level of care is needed. Modified contracts are a combination of the first two contracts and may have limits on the duration of care that can be accessed without an increase in monthly fees. Interested seniors should ask for a history of prior fee increases and detailed service charges when pursuing a CCRC investment.

Home Health

Home health care is appropriate for patients only requiring intermittent skilled services, which include nursing, physical and occupational therapy, or speech-language therapy, and further assistance may also include home health aid, behavioral health home care, and medical social work. Examples of skilled home health services include wound care for pressure sores or a surgical wound, patient and care-giver education, intravenous or nutrition therapy, injections and monitoring serious illness, and unstable health status.

Skilled nursing care will be rendered on an intermittent basis (fewer than 7 days each week or less than 8 h each day for periods of 21 days or less, with extensions in exceptional circumstances when the need for additional care is finite and predictable).

To be eligible for Medicare home health services, a patient must have Medicare Part A and/or Part B and must be homebound or confined to home. Homebound definition includes patients with disability and in constant pain.

Patient Eligibility: An individual is considered "confined to the home" (homebound) if the following two criteria are met:

First criteria	Second criteria
One of the following must be met	*Both* of the following must be met:
1. Because of illness or injury, the individual needs the aid of supportive devices such as crutches, canes, wheelchairs, and walkers; the use of special transportation; or the assistance of another person to leave their place of residence	1. There must exist a normal inability to leave home
2. Has a condition such that leaving his or her home is medically contraindicated	2. Leaving home must require a considerable and taxing effort

Per Medicare, a patient is considered homebound if absences from home are infrequent, for periods of relatively short duration, for the need to receive healthcare treatment, for religious services, to attend adult day care programs, or for other unique or infrequent events (e.g., funeral, graduation, trip to the barber).

Home health care must be furnished by or under arrangements made by a Medicare-participating home health agency (HHA). The patient must be under the care of a Medicare-enrolled physician, and the patient must receive home health services under a plan of care established and periodically reviewed by the physician without a financial relationship with the HHA. The completion of a "face-to-face encounter," related to the primary reason the patient needs home health services, is required. It can be done by the certifying physician or by a nurse practitioner or clinical nurse specialist working in collaboration with the certifying physician or a physician assistant under the supervision of the certifying physician. This encounter is required to be completed no more than 90 days prior to the home health start of care date or within 30 days of the start of the home health care.

Recertification is required after an initial 60-day period for continuous home health care unless there is patent-elected transfer or patient discharge from home health services with goals met.

Medicare does not limit the number of continuous episodes of recertification for patients who continue to be eligible for the home health benefit.

There are many home health agencies, and there are official data sets provided by the Centers for Medicare and Medicaid Services. These data allow patients to compare the quality of care provided by Medicare-certified home health agencies throughout the nation.

Home health compare is easily accessible through: www.medicare.gov/home healthcompare

Adult Day Care

Adults can receive care and companionship in adult day centers during weekdays for those who would otherwise be restrained to their homes. Preventing institutionalization and providing social activities and stimulation are underlying goals of such programs. Caregiver relief is an additional goal, enabling family caregivers to work during the day. Centers may be freestanding or located in churches or synagogues, senior centers, nursing facilities, or schools. Transportation may be available. Staff will assist with medication administration, meals, social activities, and caregiver education and counseling. If medical, nursing, or therapy services are provided on-site, it is referred to as an adult day health center. Adult day care centers are not covered by Medicare; however, Medicaid, the Veterans Administration, and the Older Americans Act may provide financial assistance. Aid for both adult day care and home caregivers through the state Departments of Aging is typically not provided.

Hospice Care

Hospice care is a philosophy of caring for the chronically ill and terminally sick with symptom management and end-of-life care, specifically addressing spiritual and emotional needs. Patients with life expectancies of 6 months or less and whose focus is on symptom management are appropriate for hospice. Hospice benefits through Medicare include medications, medical equipment, social work, nursing care, physician services, spiritual care counselors, home health aids, and bereavement services. Referrals can be made to any hospice program by the patient, family, caregiver, or physician. In the USA, hospice care is provided at patient's home, long-term facility, or an inpatient facility. Residents currently residing in a subacute or long-term care facility may enroll in hospice care at anytime; however, Medicare is unable to pay for both room and board and hospice fees. Medicaid, however, will cover room and board if you are eligible. Only medications directly related to the hospice illness will be covered by the Medicare hospice plan. Additionally, hourly care is not provided and will need to be paid for out of pocket as hospice visits are intermittent.

Care Team Members

Depending on the level of custodial care and rehabilitation provided at each senior facility, staff from multiple disciplines work together to care for each resident.

Medical Director

Medical directors are full-time or part-time licensed physicians who provide medical guidance and assist with care coordination and implementation in nursing facilities. They work with facility leadership and staff to develop and implement facility policies, making sure they are in line with current standards of care. They assist with facility quality improvement initiatives and review its MDS data and performance of the Resident Assessment Instrument (RAI) system.

Physician

Attending physicians must be familiar with the medical and psychosocial complexity of frail residents in skilled and long-term care nursing facilities. Physicians are often board certified in geriatric medicine and have a working understanding of chronic care conditions, drug prescriptions in older adults, and multidisciplinary team collaboration. They establish resident prognoses and goals; review residents' comprehensive care plans; refer for appropriate therapy, palliative care, and other specialist consultations; and ensure smooth care transitions.

Registered Nurse

Registered nurses oversee treatment at skilled and long-term care nursing facilities. The RN will supervise certified nursing assistants and licensed practical nurses and may have the title of director of nursing or head nurse. They are charged with developing resident treatment plans, delegating tasks, ensuring continuity of care, educating residents and families, and communicating with families and physicians with changes in conditions or care plans.

Licensed Practical Nurse

Licensed practical nurses (LPNs) work until the supervision of RNs or licensed physicians and provide direct bedside care. They provide personal hygiene, take vital signs, administer medications, perform wound care, and other day-to-day care. They communicate with physicians when a resident's clinical status changes or new orders have been recommended by other members of the care team.

Certified Nursing Assistant

Certified nursing assistants (CNAs) work alongside LPNs to perform activities of daily living such as bathing, toileting, transfers, and feeding. They will also assist with patient transport, linen and clothing changes, and repositioning. Unlike LPNs and RNs, they cannot administer medications, place IVs, or draw blood. CNAs must have a high school diploma or equivalent degree and be state certified.

Social Worker

The Omnibus Budget Reconciliation Act of 1987 (also called the "Nursing Home Reform Act" requires a social services director (with a masters degree in social work, bachelor's degree in social work, or bachelor's degree in a related field) for each SNF with 120 or more beds. They ensure that residents receive medically related social services, appropriate mental health interventions, and social interaction. They assist with preadmission and discharge planning, review resident rights, provide information on advanced directives, complete psychosocial components of the MDS, participate in resident care planning, and counsel residents and their families.

Physical Therapist

Physical therapists develop individual plans with residents to promote functional mobility and restore function. They can work with patients in the skilled nursing setting, in the home or as an outpatient. New patients undergo evaluations of endurance, mobility, balance, and strength. Attention is placed on bed mobility, transfers, and gait to minimize fall risk; energy conservation in those with multiple comorbid conditions; and stretching and strengthening for those who are immobilized. This is especially important for patients admitted after orthopedic surgeries.

Occupational Therapist

Occupational therapists work in collaboration with physical therapists to identify weaknesses in self-care and activities that are important to the resident. They teach functional mobility skills, such as transfers and using ambulatory devices, and enhance IADLs. They may teach compensatory techniques for those with vision, hearing, or cognitive impairment. They work with families regarding patient needs and determine what medical equipment is necessary prior to discharge from skilled nursing. They can work in program development by developing fall prevention, dementia management, repositioning, restraint reduction, and behavioral therapy programs for SNF staff.

Speech Therapist

Speech-language pathologists (SLPs) work in outpatient and inpatient settings to evaluate communication barriers due to speech, language, and cognitive impairment and swallowing disorders. SLPs must complete a masters or Ph.D. degree and an additional 9-month fellowship under direct supervision. It is expected that by 2020 the SLP job market will grow by more than 20 % to meet the demands of the growing senior population [17]. Their work with stroke victims (75 % of which occur in adults 65 years and older), patients with Alzheimer's disease (who commonly develop language disturbances), and Parkinson's patients (often burdened by dysphagia and dementia) is critical in optimizing daily communication skills. For those with cognitive impairment, SLPs can perform home visits to provide caregiver training, make environmental modifications, and recommend routine and activity alterations.

Dietician

Dieticians evaluate residents with weight loss or gain, wounds or skin breakdown, and those with serum markers of malnutrition. After meeting with residents upon admission to develop a plan of care, they make recommendations for diets, food restrictions, and supplements to the physician for approval. They may also assess food preparation and handling at skilled nursing facilities and assist in management of the food budget.

Caregivers

"Nonmedical" or "unskilled" care is performed by CNAs, home health aids (HHAs), or personal care aids (PCAs) who work under a state-licensed agency. Some states are now requiring an hourly minimal of training for in-home caregivers, ranging from 40 to 100 h. Home caregivers must be supervised by a registered nurse who performs an initial assessment and develops the plan of care. Unskilled caregiver services include custodial and hygienic care. They may perform homemaker tasks such as meal preparation, errands, light housework, and transportation services. Services are provided in 4-h increments, up to 24 h/day, or as a bed and bathing service in which the caregiver makes nightly visits to assist with bedtime activities. Unskilled care is paid for privately or less commonly by Medicaid pending eligibility. Medicare will not cover unskilled care, but will pay for *skilled care* if a patient is homebound; requires intermittent nursing care, physical therapy, or speech therapy; and has an order from their physician.

Care Facility Summary [18]

The choice for the discharge destination will depend on the needs of the elder patient and the services available at each setting.

Care settings	Synonyms	Overview	Physician type	Requirements for admission	Coverage	Cost
Acute rehabilitation	Acute inpatient rehabilitation	Special hospital unit offering intense PT and OT	Physiatrist	Physician request. Patient must be able to tolerate 3 h of therapy daily and show progress to continue coverage through Medicare	Medicare Part A (hospital insurance)—coverage of 100 days of stay with qualifying diagnosis; Medicaid	$1000–2000/day
Subacute rehabilitation (SAR)	Skilled nursing facility (SNF)	Nursing home providing care post-hospitalization, certified through Medicare	Geriatrician, nurse practitioner, physician's assistant, medical director	Patient must have skilled need (IV medication, wound care, rehabilitation)	Medicare, Medicaid	$150–300/day
Long-term acute care (LTAC)	Transitional care hospital, "chronic hospitalization"	Facility	Hospitalist, intensivist	Require complex care; ventilator care, and weaning	Medicare	$1500–3000/day
Nursing home	Long-term care	Custodial care	Geriatrician	Require assistance with custodial, skilled, and/or non-skilled care	Medicaid in some states	$75–300/day
Assisted living (AL)	Residential care, board and care, adult care home, adult group home	Institutional care in private living quarters; heterogeneous services typically include meals, medication management, and housekeeping	Primary care physician	Less disabled than nursing homes. Require some personal care services but not 24-h supervision	Medicaid in some states, supplemental security, VA, long-term insurance, private PA	$60–300/day
Independent living (IL)	Retirement homes, retirement communities, senior housing	Housing arrangement for adults 55 years and older offering amenities, activities, and services	Primary care physician	Must require little or no assistance with ADLs as medical care or nursing staff is typically not offered on-site	Private pay, long-term insurance with home care benefits	$50–100/day

			Multidisciplinary team	Health screening		
Continuing care retirement community (CCRC)	Life care communities	Retirement community that offers several levels of care on the same grounds, enabling patients to transfer between them as their needs change			Entrance fee followed by monthly fees	Entrance fee: $100,000–$1,000,000 Monthly fee: $3000–$5000
Unskilled home health care	Home caregiver, homemaker, home health aid	ADL and IADL assistance in-home setting; bed and bathing services	CNA, home health aid; supervised by RN	No criteria	Private pay, Medicaid, long-term care insurance	$8–40/h typically in 4-h blocks; average $20/h
Skilled home health care	Home health care	Nursing care, therapy visits (PT, OT, ST), patient education, home safety evaluation, SW support	RN or LPN	Homebound, require intermittent nursing care or therapy services, under regular care of a physician	Medicare Part A and/or Part B, private insurance	$100–300/h
Adult day care	Adult day health center	Nonresidential care center providing social support, recreational services, ADL assistance, and caregiver relief	SW, RN; may have PT, OT, ST, MD, mental health, dietician if an adult day health center	Cannot safely be left alone; needs structure in day; primary caregiver must work outside of the home	Private pay, Medicaid, Veterans Administration	$25–100/day
End-of-life care	Hospice care	Provides end-of-life care through symptom and pain management support during dying process and bereavement period	Interprofessional team providing care at home, inpatient setting, or skilled nursing facility	Life expectancy is 6 months or less; must be recertified by a physician each benefit period	Medicare, Medicaid, private insurance	Generally provided without charge

Other Items to Understand About Subacute Rehabilitation/ Skilled Nursing Facilities

Minimum Data Set

All residents in a Medicare- or Medicaid-certified nursing facility undergo a federally mandated process of screening and clinical assessment upon admission to the facility and, periodically, within specific guidelines and time frames. This interdisciplinary and individualized assessment, intended to serve as the basis for the plan of care, is referred to as the RAI, and one of the components of this instrument is the MDS (http://www.cms.gov/Medicare/Quality-Initiatives-Patient-Assessment-Instruments/NursingHomeQualityInits/MDS30RAIManual.html). The MDS contains items that measure physical, psychological, and psychosocial functioning. The items in the MDS give a multidimensional view of the patient's functional capacities and help staff to identify health problems. The instrument is divided in sections A through Z and has 450 items addressing clinical and functional aspects of the resident such as physical functioning, cognition, sensory, oral health, nutrition, skin, elimination, mobility, clinical conditions, or diseases. As a screening tool, it indicates the problem but it does not determine the cause of it. The resource available to assist nurses to do further assessments specific to the identified problem (such as dehydration or constipation, for instance) is the Care Area Assessment process, another component of the RAI. In a nutshell, the RAI process drives the care plan that is developed for the resident.

The MDS assessment is completed for all residents in certified nursing facilities, regardless of source of payment for the individual resident. It is, at a minimum, reassessed on a quarterly basis or whenever there is a significant change in the resident's condition. Nursing facilities may or may not maintain a hard copy version of the MDS in the resident's chart. In any instance, access to the electronic version of the MDS should be readily available to the multidisciplinary team.

The information collected in the MDS is electronically transmitted by the nursing facility to the MDS database in the respective state. The MDS information from the state databases is then captured into the national MDS database at the Centers for Medicare and Medicaid Services (CMS).

The information filled out on the MDS determines the Resource Utilization Group (RUG) category, which ultimately determines the per diem rate paid to the facility for a resident whose stay is covered under Medicare Part A.

Gradual Dose Reductions

The management of behavioral disorders in post-hospital care settings can be quite challenging whether the behavior issue stems from dementia or another chronic mental illness. Psychotropic medication misuse in older adults can lead to frequent and serious adverse outcomes and worsening of cognition and overall medical condition. In an effort to minimize this problem, the nursing home reform legislation,

Omnibus Budget Reconciliation Act of 1987 (OBRA-87), mandates that residents in nursing facilities should be free from medically unnecessary "physical or chemical restraints imposed for purposes of discipline or convenience." With this in mind, the measurement of restraint use is a CMS (Centers for Medicare and Medicaid Services) quality indicator. Post-acute care facilities have, for the most part, limited ability to manage behavioral problems and often will exclude admission of a symptomatic hospitalized patient.

Nonetheless, the prevalence of such agents in post-acute care is significant. In one nationwide study of 16,586 newly admitted residents to nursing homes, more than 29 % of subjects received at least one antipsychotic medication, and of those users, 32 % had no identified clinical indication for this therapy [19].

The prevalence of the use of antipsychotic medications is a CMS quality indicator for both short- and long-term SNF (skilled nursing facility) residents.

Significant changes took place in the survey guidance of the State Operations Manual related to the gradual dose reduction and tapering of medications with an emphasis on the importance of seeking an appropriate dose and duration for each medication.

Drug Formularies

Skilled nursing facilities each work with one pharmacy to meet the pharmaceutical needs of their patients. Upon admission, the physician will be contacted to verify the patient's medications. These orders are then faxed to the pharmacy, which will deliver the medications within 6–12 h. "STAT" (urgent or rush) medications may still take 6 h to arrive; therefore, each SNF has an emergency medication box containing antihypertensives, antipsychotics, and medications for symptom management, with only several pills of stocked controlled substances. Convenience boxes (C-boxes) may also be on-site and stocked with routinely used medications per request of the nursing facility. It is recommended that the sending physician will include scripts for schedule II and III medications with the patient, as pharmacies will fill narcotic medications ordered over the phone only in emergency situations. Each pharmacy will have a unique formulary; therefore, patients may be transitioned to alternate medications in the same class if appropriate. Formularies are utilized to lower costs, facilitate quicker delivery, and enhance safety by increasing nurse familiarity with provided medications.

Ancillary Services

Ancillary services such a blood draws and portable images may be performed at nursing homes. Imaging services typically include X-rays, ultrasounds including venous duplexes, and electrocardiograms. Portable imaging suppliers travel to facilities as needed, typically within 24 h. Laboratory specimens including urine samples and serum blood tests can be collected by in-house nurses or an outside laboratory phlebotomist; however, these services may not be offered on weekends. Peripheral IVs and PICC line placements, initiation of nasogastric tube feedings, urinary catheter placement, staple and suture removal, and wound care are available at skilled nursing facilities. Procedures or tests that must be performed within 30–60 min will require transfer to the local emergency department. Transfusions, IV chemotherapy, hemodialysis, BiPAP initiation, continuous telemetry, and minor surgeries are typically not performed at SNFs.

Key Points
1. Older adults have a number of options for post-hospitalization care that include acute inpatient rehabilitation (AIR), long-term acute care hospital (LTACH), subacute rehabilitation (skilled nursing facility—SNF), independent and assisted living facilities, continuing care retirement community (CCRC), home health (skilled and unskilled), adult day care, and hospice care.
2. Physicians are increasingly asked for their viewpoint on what is the best post-hospitalization care setting for the older adult patient and need to be aware of the nuances of each.
3. Determining the post-hospitalization needs of the older adult is the best place to start in deciding on a discharged location.
4. Resources are available to select the optimal post-hospitalization care facility which are publicly accessible (e.g., Medicare.gov/nursinghomecompare or eldercare locator).
5. Multidisciplinary teams work at most post-acute facilities, and understanding the responsibilities of each role is important for clinicians, patients, and families.
6. Mandated by Medicare of skilled nursing/subacute rehabilitation facilities, gradual dose reductions of antipsychotic medications must be regularly attempted for all residents or reasons for exceptions formally written in the patients' charts.
7. Each facility may have their own pharmacy, either off-site or in building, and the medication formulary may differ between hospital and facility.

References

1. Boockvar KS, et al. Patient relocation in the 6 months after hip fracture: risk factors for fragmented care. J Am Geriatr Soc. 2004;52(11):1826–31.
2. Horwitz LI, et al. Transfers of patient care between house staff on internal medicine wards: a national survey. Arch Intern Med. 2006;166(11):1173–7.
3. Ward KT, et al. Do internal medicine residents know enough about skilled nursing facilities to orchestrate a good care transition? J Am Med Dir Assoc. 2014;15(11):841–3.
4. Kane RL. Finding the right level of post hospital care: "We didn't realize there was any other option for him". JAMA. 2011;305(3):284–93.
5. Ouslander JG, Lamb G, Perloe M, et al. Potentially avoidable hospitalizations of nursing home residents: frequency, causes, and costs. J Am Geriatr Soc. 2010;58(4):627–35. 760–1.
6. Katz S, Ford AB, Moskowitz RW, Jackson BA, Jaffe MW. Studies of illness in the aged: the index of ADL: a standardized measure of biological and psychosocial function. JAMA. 1963;185(12):914–9.

7. Mahoney FI, Barthel DW. Functional evaluation: the Barthel Index. Md State Med J. 1965;14:61–5.
8. Lawton MP, Brody EM. Assessment of older people: self-maintaining and instrumental activities of daily living. Gerontologist. 1969;9(3):179–86.
9. Folstein MF, Folstein SE, McHugh PR. "Mini-mental state"; a practical method for grading the cognitive state of patients for the clinician. J Psychiatr Res. 1975;12(3):189–98.
10. Berstein IH, Lacritz L, Barlow CF, Weiner MF, DeFina LF. Psychometric evaluation of the Montreal Cognitive Assessment (MoCA) in three diverse samples. Clin Neuropsychol. 2011;25(1):119–26.
11. Borson S, Scanlan JM, Chen P, Ganguli M. The Mini-Cog as a screen for dementia: validation in a population-based sample. JAGS. 2003;51(10):1451–4.
12. Inouye S, van Dyck C, Alessi C, Balkin S, Siegal A, Horwitz R. Clarifying confusion: the confusion assessment method. Ann Intern Med. 1990;113(12):941–8.
13. Podsiadlo D, Richardson S. The timed "Up and Go": a test of basic functional mobility for frail elderly persons. J Am Geriatr Soc. 1991;39:142–8.
14. Nursing Home Compare. Medicare.gov Website. 2015. http://www.medicare.gov/NHCompare/Include? dataSection/Questions?SearchCriteriaNEW.asp. Accessed 13 June 2015.
15. 2015 Medicare & You. National Medicare Handbook. Centers for Medicare & Medicaid Services, Baltimore, MD, 2014.
16. Dworkin A (2010) Oregon among national leaders in number of assisted living facilities. Oregonian. http://www.oregonlive.com/news/index.ssf/2010/01/oregon_among_national_leaders.html.
17. Bureau of Labor Statistics, U.S. Department of Labor. Occupational outlook handbook, 2012–13 edition, Speech–Language Pathologists. http://www.bls.gov/ooh/healthcare/speech-language-pathologists.htm.
18. Genworth 2015 Cost of Care Survey. 2015. https://www.genworth.com/dam/Americas/US/PDFs/Consumer/corporate/130568_040115_gnw.pdf.
19. Chen Y, et al. Unexplained variation across US nursing homes in antipsychotic prescribing rates. Arch Intern Med. 2010;170(1):89–95.

Utilizing Geriatric Assessments to Fulfill the Medicare Annual Wellness Visits

Ming Jang, Rachel K. Miller, and Lee A. Lindquist

The population of older adults, aged 65 years and older, reached 46.2 million in 2014 and is projected to more than double to 80 million by 2050 [1]. Advances in healthcare have enabled patients to live longer with less functional disabilities [2]. When an older adult presents for an annual checkup, most of the clinical time is spent on managing the progression of chronic health issues and evaluating acute symptoms in an aging body. Besides these issues, completing a geriatric assessment can be very helpful in uncovering life-impacting problems, which many patients may not even realize is happening to them. A frequent misconception among patients is that many problems are due to "old age" and not fixable. It takes a meticulous physician to check older adults for geriatric issues and find remedies that frequently improve the older adult's quality of life.

The comprehensive geriatric assessment (CGA) has been a mainstay of geriatrics care and clinical education [3]. Involving a myriad of assessments and system reviews, the CGA can establish a baseline for the aging patient's clinical status as well as uncover patient's specific needs [4]. The diversity of these needs is as broad as the spectrum of patients that end up needing care. It is therefore important that the clinicians be comfortable in conducting a comprehensive geriatric evaluation, assessing for various environmental risk factors, and screening for medication nonadherence, caregiver burnout, or malnutrition risk.

M. Jang (✉) • R.K. Miller
Division of Geriatrics, Perelman School of Medicine, Hospital of the University of Pennsylvania, Philadelphia, PA, USA

L.A. Lindquist
Division of General Internal Medicine and Geriatrics, Northwestern University Feinberg School of Medicine, Chicago, IL, USA
e-mail: LAL425@md.northwestern.edu

© Springer International Publishing Switzerland 2016
L.A. Lindquist (ed.), *New Directions in Geriatric Medicine*,
DOI 10.1007/978-3-319-28137-7_10

The Comprehensive Geriatric Assessment

There are many versions of this assessment available—each one catered to specific provider preferences. However, the spirit of the CGA remains constant throughout and is composed of the following aspects:

1. *Functional Assessment*: At the heart of the CGA lies the functional assessment. A useful tool for tabulating the level of basic and instrumental activities of daily living (ADL) dependency is the Katz ADL and Lawton independent ADL score, respectively [5, 6]. Besides ADL evaluations, measuring the gait speed can predict functional decline and early mortality in older adults [7].
2. *Cognitive Assessment*: For the busy clinician, a Mini-Cog exam (three-word recall and clock draw) is a quick, reasonable, sensitive, and specific screen to tease out concern for cognitive impairment [8]. For those who screen positive for cognitive impairment, a more detailed examination like the Montreal Cognitive Assessment (MOCA) or the Short Portable Mental Status Questionnaire (SPMSQ) can be administered [9, 10].
3. *Depression Screening*: The USPSTF recommends depression screening for all older adults if the appropriate interventional resources are in place [11, 12]. Specific to older adults, the Geriatric Depression Scale exists in both a short form (15 items) and long form (30 items) [13]. Also effective in identifying depression, the Patient Health Questionnaire—9 or 2 (PHQ-9, PHQ-2)—is shorter and sometimes preferred by busy clinicians [14, 15]. A positive screen for either of these tests requires further investigation or discussion.
4. *Vision*: It is reasonable to query patients about a history of vision changes. Most patients experience worsening vision and rely on eyewear to see as they age. It is a worthwhile question to ask how old their glasses are or when was the last time that their vision has been evaluated. In evaluating vision, a Snellen pocket chart is an inexpensive, simple tool to use for such occasions. Patients with a history of diabetes, or have high risk of glaucoma, should have yearly evaluations [16].
5. *Hearing*: Hearing loss is often missed by patients but can be readily identified by their neighbors, telephone partners, or loved ones. It remains reasonable to ask for a history of hearing loss or to base your concern on clinical suspicion. Ruling out cerumen impaction with an otoscope is important prior to arranging an audiology evaluation. One should keep in mind that cerumen impaction contributing to hearing loss can be mistaken for cognitive loss in the older adults [17, 18].
6. *Dentition*: It is useful to be aware of pending dental emergencies or oral manifestation of systemic illnesses. Poor dentition should be noted, along with the proper fitting of dentures or assistive devices. Mucositis, gingivitis, buccal cellulitis/abscess, and oral ulcers should be assessed if there's a specific oral concern. Loose teeth should be noted and the patient referred to dentistry, as this is a risk for tooth aspiration [19].

7. *Nutritional Assessment*: Older adults are at high risk for multifactorial malnutrition and weight loss. In addition, specific nutrient deficiencies can compound and present as certain geriatric syndromes. Asking patients about their food and drink intake and quantifying the amount is a quick start. Another quick check is looking at the waistband or fit of their clothes. If the patient has lost weight in their midsection, it will be apparent by the belt holes or gap between skin and pants. The Nutritional Health Checklist and Mini Nutritional Assessment are simple tools that can be used to screen at-risk older adults [20–22]. A positive screen would indicate that the patient is at a high nutritional risk, necessitating further investigation into the potential cause and resultant interventions.

8. *Urinary and Fecal Incontinence*: Bowel incontinence and bladder incontinence have a significant impact on institutionalization and contribute to morbidity and mortality [23]. Important medical repercussions also include infections, renal failure, and sepsis [24, 25]. The history and physical should try to differentiate the type of incontinence which then allows the clinician to tailor the intervention.

9. *Balance and Falls*: Falls remain a significant contributor to Medicare costs and overall patient morbidity and mortality. For those who have fallen, the subsequent fear of falling then contributes to this vicious syndrome. The Timed Get Up and Go Test is a useful tool to screen for fall risk as is the Tinetti Balance and Gait Evaluation [26]. Addressing the patients' intrinsic and extrinsic risk factors, considering osteoporosis screening/treatment, reevaluating need for anticoagulation if patient is on it, and mobilizing therapy resources are all appropriate interventions.

10. *Osteoporosis Screening*: The USPSTF recommends all females aged 65 and older to have bone density screening [27]. There are no recommendations for osteoporosis screening in men. However, those who have risk factors for osteoporosis should be considered as candidates for screening [28].

11. *Polypharmacy*: Most older adults take multiple medications, with some patients taking over ten medications [29]. Pill burden, inaccurate medication lists, pharmacologic interactions, metabolism changes, and sensitivity/ adverse reactions to side effects work together to worsen outcomes in at-risk patients. At each visit, a medication reconciliation should be done with the patient or their care provider, and BEERS listed medications should be considered for removal. The medications contained on the BEERS list medications are considered to be potentially harmful to adults as they age [30]. In addition, older adults receive multiple directions on how to take their medications (e.g., from physicians, nurses, home nurses, pharmacists, pill bottles). Evidence has shown that older adults frequently unnecessarily overcomplicate their medication regimens. Patients may take medications before or after meals, wake up at 11 p.m. to take a medication slotted for bedtime, or rise at 5 a.m. to take a morning medication. Clinicians can simplify their medication regimen easily by inquiring "Walk me through your day—tell me how you take your medications" [31].

12. *Screening for Cancer*
    (a) *Lung*: Routine screening has not yet been advised. Low-dose CT imaging may be obtained in the right clinical scenario at any point.
    (b) *Prostate*: There are various recommendations depending on the specialty. Many geriatricians believe that there is over testing and over·treatment. This screening should be done as a case by case basis.
    (c) *Cervical*: The USPSTF recommends screening for cervical cancer for women aged 21–65; however, the evidence is inconclusive on whether to continue screening over the age of 65 years. There are more structured recommendations from ACOG, who recommend that women over age 65 with three consecutive negative pap smears do not require additional screening. It is reasonable to consider each patient separately but consider stopping screening for those older than age 65 years who have had adequate prior screening and are not otherwise at high risk for cervical cancer.
    (d) *Colon*: The age to initiate colon cancer screening is concrete, but there is no specified cutoff age. The general idea is that if the patient is highly functional and is in the middle to upper tier of physical health compared to their sicker same-age peers, they may benefit from continued colon cancer screening.
    (e) *Breast*: Initial age of screening is less concrete than with colon cancer screening. However, by the time patients enter the older adult population, they usually will have multiple mammograms. Continuing screening mammography for patients as they age will have to occur on the case by case basis, but generally, like with colon cancer patients, the patient with shorter life expectancy may not benefit from the investigation and treatment. The US Preventive Services Task Force (USPSTF) recommends that women aged 50–69 receive timely breast cancer screening but does not make a recommendation for women aged 70 and older [32–34].

13. *Psychosocial Environment*: Knowing a patient's social and family support structures is a vital step in allowing the clinician to provide patient-centered care. Place of birth, religion/spirituality, level of education, military service, present and prior marriages, involved family/friends, and community/religious activities are all important pieces of information. The presence of decision makers should be elucidated as well and whether or not these players are designated medical or financial power of attorneys. Functioning utilities is also of critical note. Home and gun ownership is relevant as well, along with the presence of stairs and number of levels to the home. Additionally, knowing which floor the bedroom is on, and the bathroom, is important especially for patients at risk for falling. Lastly, financial security should be assessed and the presence of accessory support structures.

14. *End-of-Life Wishes and Code Status*: Determining a patient's code status and wishes for end of life is important. If not completed, introducing who would be the patient's power of attorney is vital in the event that the patient ever needs to have a surrogate decision maker [35].

A major concern with conducting a CGA is the sheer amount of time it entails, frequently lasting forty minutes or longer. Historically, the Medicare reimbursements for CGAs have been lacking. However, in recent years, payments for the Medicare Annual Wellness Visits have been instituted and allow for a higher reimbursement for clinicians. Many of the requirements for the Medicare Annual Wellness Visits can be accounted for by the components of the CGA.

Meeting the Needs of the Medicare Annual Wellness Visit Through Adaptation of the CGA

The Medicare Modernization Act (MMA) authorized full payment for an Initial Preventive Physical Examination (IPPE), also known as the "Welcome to Medicare Preventive Visit," beginning in 2005 (https://www.medicare.gov/coverage/preventive-visit-and-yearly-wellness-exams.html). This legislation also provided payment for a follow-up Annual Wellness Visit (AWV) every 12 months to continue to monitor and build upon the plan created as part of the IPPE. The intention of these visits is to provide patients and physicians a means of completing a comprehensive well-being and preventative care evaluation. Clinicians can be motivated to conduct these types of visits as they are not only good care for patients but are also being reimbursed at higher rates than the average outpatient visit. Clinicians are not the only ones who may benefit financially. Several insurers, who provide Medicare coverage, have begun to offer patients financial incentives (e.g., $75 gift cards, coupons) for having the IPPE or AWV completed.

Operationalizing the Medicare Wellness Visits may seem overwhelming at first. However, when a framework is built according to individual practice needs, completing and billing for the Medicare Wellness Visits is workable. In practices that use electronic health records, shortcuts, prompts, or preconfigured forms (e.g., SmartSets) can be used to complete these types of visits.

Besides the routine parts of an office visit (e.g., vitals, exam, diagnoses, plan), parts from the CGA can be used to fulfill the needs of the Medicare Annual Wellness Visit. The main components necessary for the Medicare Wellness Visits and possible means of completing them are as in Table 10.1.

In addition to these components, there are a number of other Medicare Part B preventive services that qualify under the Annual Wellness Visits. Included are screening for osteoporosis, cardiovascular disease, breast/prostate/colon cancer, diabetes, HIV, and hepatitis C; counseling to stop alcohol misuse and tobacco use; and vaccination administration for influenza, pneumococcal, and hepatitis B vaccinations.

While rules frequently change as to what is covered or required in documentation, the Centers for Medicare and Medicaid Services website (available at www.cms.gov) can provide clinicians with the most up-to-date recommendations for the Medicare Annual Wellness Visit.

Table 10.1 Medicare Annual Wellness Visit and components of CGA

Past medical/surgical history—including hospitalizations and allergies	
Current medications—including over-the-counter medications, supplements, and vitamins	
Family history	
Tobacco use	
Alcohol use	
Illicit drug use	
Exercise and physical activity	
Diet	Nutritional assessments
Review for potential risk factors for depression and mood disorders	
Depression screening	PHQ-2, PHQ-9, GDS
Review of functional ability and level of safety	
Hearing impairment	Whisper test, audiometer
Vision difficulty	Snellen chart
Activities of daily living assessment	Katz ADLS/IADLS, gait speed
Fall risk	Timed get up and go
Home safety	Asking the question: is there anything about living at home that makes you feel unsafe?
End-of-life planning/advance planning	

Key Points

1. For patients aged 65 years and older, a clinician should review for geriatric issues occurring and can utilize the comprehensive geriatric assessment (CGA) as a tool.
2. Older adults may be unaware that they are experiencing senior-specific issues and that these issues can be remedied.
3. The CGA varies by user and institution but primarily encompasses screening for function, memory, depression, vision, hearing, dental, nutrition, incontinence, balance, polypharmacy, cancer screening, and end of life.
4. The CGA can be time consuming but recent changes in Medicare reimbursement allows for preventative Wellness Visits which have requirements that overlap with the CGA.
5. Completing a Medicare Wellness Visit and/or CGA can be exceptionally helpful for older adults to age successfully and engage in a healthy active life.

References

1. Werner C, U.S. Census Brief. The older population: 2010. United States Census Bureau. November 2011. Available at https://www.census.gov/prod/cen2010/briefs/c2010br-09.pdf.
2. Statistical Brief. Sixty-five plus in the United States, United States Census Bureau. Economics and Statistics Administration, U.S. Department of Commerce. May 1995. Available at https://www.census.gov/population/socdemo/statbriefs/agebrief.html.
3. Stuck AE, Siu AL, Wieland GD, Adams JL, Rubenstein LZ. Comprehensive geriatric assessment: a meta-analysis of controlled trials. Lancet. 1993;342:1032–6.

4. Kuo HK, Scandrett KG, Dave J, Mitchell SL. The influence of outpatient comprehensive geriatric assessment on survival: a meta-analysis. Arch Gerontol Geriatr. 2004;39:245.
5. Katz S, Downs TD, Cash HR, Grotz RC. Progress in development of the index of ADL. Gerontologist. 1970;10:20–30.
6. Lawton MP, Brody EM. Assessment of older people: self-maintaining and instrumental activities of daily living. Gerontologist. 1969;9:179–86.
7. Studenski S, Perera S, Patel K, Rosano C, Faulkner K, Inzitari M, Brach J, Chandler J, Cawthon P, Connor EB, Nevitt M, Visser M, Kritchevsky S, Badinelli S, Harris T, Newman AB, Cauley J, Ferrucci L. Guralnik. Gait speed and survival in older adults. JAMA. 2011;305(1):50.
8. Borson S, Scanlan J, Brush M, Vitaliano P, Dokmak A. The Mini-Cog: a cognitive "vital sign" measure for dementia screening in multi-lingual eldelr. Int J Geriatr Psychiatry. 2000;15(11): 1021–7.
9. Pfeiffer E. A short portable mental status questionnaire for the assessment of organic brain deficit in elderly patients. J Am Geriatr Soc. 1975;23(10):433–41.
10. Nasreddine ZS, Phillips NA, Bedirian V, Charbonneau S, Whitehead V, Collin I, et al. The Montreal Cognitive Assessment, MoCA: a brief screening tool for mild cognitive impairment. J Am Geriatr Soc. 2005;53:695–9. http://www.mocatest.org/.
11. O'Connor EA, Whitlock EP, Gaynes B, Beil TL. Screening for depression in adults and older adults in primary care: an updated systematic review. Evidence Synthesis No. 75. Rockville: Agency for Healthcare Research and Quality; 2009. (AHRQ Publication No. 10-05143-EF-1).
12. US Preventive Services Task Force. Services Task Force. Screening for depression: recommendations and rationale. Ann Intern Med. 2002;136:760–4.
13. Sheikh JI, Yesavage JA. Geriatric depression scale: recent evidence and development of a shorter version. Clin Gerontol. 1986;5:165–72.
14. Kroenke K, Spitzer RL, Williams JB. The PHQ-9: validity of a brief depression severity measure. J Gen Intern Med. 2001;16:606.
15. Arroll B, Khin N, Kerse N. Screening for depression in primary care with two verbally asked questions: cross sectional study. BMJ. 2003;327:1144.
16. Crews JE, Campbell VA. Vision impairment and hearing loss among community-dwelling older americans: implications for health and functioning. Am J Public Health. 2004;94(5):823–9.
17. Moore AM, Voytas J, Kowalski D, Maddens M. Cerumen, hearing, and cognition in the elderly. J Am Med Dir Assoc. 2002;3(3):136–9.
18. Oron Y, Zwecker-Lazar I, Levy D, Kreitler S, Roth Y. Cerumen removal: comparison of cerumenolytic agents and effect on cognition among the elderly. Arch Gerontol Geriatr. 2011;52(2):228–32. doi:10.1016/j.archger.2010.03.025.
19. Vargas CM, Kramarow EA, Yellowitz JA. The oral health of older Americans, Aging Trends, No. 3. Hyattsville: National Center for Health Statistics; 2001.
20. Ranhoff AH, Gjøen AU, Mowé M. Screening for malnutrition in elderly acute medical patients: the usefulness of MNA-SF. J Nutr Health Aging. 2005;9(4):221–5.
21. Guigoz Y, Lauque S, Vellas BJ. Identifying the elderly at risk for malnutrition. The Mini Nutritional Assessment. Clin Geriatr Med. 2002;18(4):737–57.
22. de Groot LC, Beck AM, Schroll M, van Staveren WA. Evaluating the DETERMINE Your Nutritional Health Checklist and the Mini Nutritional Assessment as tools to identify nutritional problems in elderly Europeans. Eur J Clin Nutr. 1998;52(12):877–83.
23. Brandeis GH, Baumann MM, Hossain M, et al. The prevalence of potentially remediable urinary incontinence in frail older people: a study using the Minimum Data Set. J Am Geriatr Soc. 1997;45:179.
24. Fung CH, Spencer B, Eslami M, Crandall C. Quality indicators for the screening and care of urinary incontinence in vulnerable elders. J Am Geriatr Soc. 2007;55 Suppl 2:S443.
25. Roberts RO, Jacobsen SJ, Rhodes T, et al. Urinary incontinence in a community-based cohort: prevalence and healthcare-seeking. J Am Geriatr Soc. 1998;46:467.
26. Lachs MS, Feinstein AR, Cooney Jr LM, Drickamer MA, Marottoli RA, Pannill FC, Tinetti ME. A simple procedure for general screening for functional disability in elderly patients. Ann Intern Med. 1990;112(9):699–706.

27. U.S. Preventive Services Task Force. Final update summary: osteoporosis: screening. U.S. Preventive Services Task Force. 2015. http://www.uspreventiveservicestaskforce.org/Page/Document/UpdateSummaryFinal/osteoporosis-screening
28. Rao SS, Budhwar N, Ashfaque A. Osteoporosis in men. Am Fam Physician. 2010;82(5):503–8.
29. Willlams CM. Using medications appropriately in older adults. Am Fam Physician. 2002;66:1917.
30. American Geriatrics Society 2012 Beers Criteria Update Expert Panel. American geriatrics society updated beers criteria for potentially inappropriate medication use in older adults. J Am Geriatr Soc. 2012;60:616.
31. Lindquist LA, Lindquist LM, Zickuhr L, Friesema E, Wolf MS. Unnecessary complexity of home medication regimens among seniors. Patient Educ Couns. 2014;96(1):93–7.
32. Schonberg MA, McCarthy EP, Davis RB, Phillips RS, Hamel MB. Breast cancer screening in women aged 80 and older: results from a national survey. J Am Geriatr Soc. 2004;52(10): 1688–95.
33. Caplan LS. To screen or not to screen: the issue of breast cancer screening in older women. Public Health Rev. 2001;29(2-4):231–40.
34. Blustein J, Weiss LJ. The use of mammography by women aged 75 and older: factors related to health, functioning, and age. J Am Geriatr Soc. 1998;46(8):941–6.
35. Sudore RL, Fried TR. Redefining the "planning" in advance care planning: preparing for end-of-life decision making. Ann Intern Med. 2010;153:256.

Index

© Springer International Publishing Switzerland 2016
L.A. Lindquist (ed.), *New Directions in Geriatric Medicine*,
DOI 10.1007/978-3-319-28137-7